CRITICAL ISSUES IN SURGERY

CRITICAL ISSUES IN SURGERY

Edited by

Aurel C. Cernaianu
Anthony J. DelRossi
and
Richard K. Spence

University of Medicine and Dentistry of New Jersey
Robert Wood Johnson Medical School at Camden
Camden, New Jersey

SPRINGER SCIENCE+BUSINESS MEDIA, LLC

Library of Congress Cataloging-in-Publication Data

On file

Proceedings of the First and Second Annual Meetings on Critical Issues in Surgery,
held November 1992 and November 1993 (respectively),
in St. Thomas, U. S. Virgin Islands

ISBN 978-0-306-44918-5   ISBN 978-1-4615-1851-8 (eBook)
DOI 10.1007/978-1-4615-1851-8

© 1995 Springer Science+Business Media New York
Originally published by Plenum Press in 1995

PREFACE

The topics in this book represent the presentations given at the First and Second Annual Meetings entitled "Critical Issues in Surgery" held at the Frenchman's Reef Beach Resort, St. Thomas, U.S. Virgin Islands, November 1992 and 1993.

This symposium was sponsored by the Department of Surgery, and the Department of Nursing Education and Quality Assurance of Cooper Hospital/University Medical Center, the University of Medicine and Dentistry of New Jersey, Robert Wood Johnson Medical School, Camden, New Jersey, as well as the Academy of Medicine of New Jersey.

Chapter authors were charged with the task of writing brief overviews of major issues related to the field of general surgery and critical care medicine. The book is specifically tailored to the needs of general surgeons, allied health professionals and nursing personnel involved in all phases of caring for the surgical patient.

Although intended as a reference source with emphasis on up-dated approaches applied in general surgery, it is hoped that the discussion of these topics will compliment other texts and manuscripts. Obviously, a book of this length cannot cover the whole multidisciplinary and complex field of surgery. However, the co-editors are certain that the annual appearance of this text will highlight comprehensive, new and interesting approaches to the field of surgery.

The co-editors are greatly thankful to the contributors for their efforts in providing comprehensive chapters. Without their expertise, this work may not have been possible. We would also like to thank Ms. Mary Safford, Eileen Bermingham and the staff at Plenum Publishing Corporation for their tremendous help in completing this work.

Aurel C. Cernaianu, M.D.
Anthony J. DelRossi, M.D.
Richard K. Spence, M.D.

CONTENTS

The Role of Nutrition in Wound Healing   1
    Stanley J. Dudrick, M.D.

Chronic Wounds: Growth Factors and Comprehensive Surgical Care . . . 13
    David R. Knighton, M.D.

Wound Healing and Infection 25
    Donald E. Fry, M.D.

The *Plug* Repair for Recurrent Inguinal Hernias 33
    Alex G. Shulman, M.D.

Open Tension-Free Repair of Primary Inguinal Hernias in Adult Males 41
    Alex G. Shulman, M.D.

Sepsis and Its Related Disorders: Definitions, Epidemiology,
    Pathogenesis and Pathophysiology 51
    Bruce Friedman, M.D.

The Septic Patient: Future Directions 63
    T. James Gallagher, M.D.

Prophylaxis and Therapeutic Clinical Trials in Severe Sepsis and
    Septic Shock 69
    Gus J. Slotman, M.D.

Pharmacologic Management of Postoperative Infections 77
    Jacqueline D. Sutton, Pharm.D.

The Resuscitation Game 89
    Mary McCarthy, M.D.

Transfusion Guidelines for Elective Surgery: The Transfusion Trigger 95
    Richard K. Spence, M.D.

Physiologic Predictors of Transfusion Need in the Intensive Care Unit 103
    Loren D. Nelson, M.D.

Preoperative Autologous Blood Donation 123
    Lawrence T. Goodnough, MD

Component Therapy 131
    Keith F. O'Malley, M.D.

The Anesthesiologist's Viewpoint: Transfusion, Hemodilution and
    Cooperation 137
    Linda Stehling, M.D.

Endovascular Surgery 145
    Sushil K. Gupta, M.D., Nissage Cadet, M.D., and Thomas K.
    Whang, M.D.

Hypomagnesemia as a Predictor of Mortality in Critically Ill Trauma
    Patients 153
    Philip C. Wry, M.D., Anthony J. Mure, M.D., and Steven E. Ross,
    M.D.

Abdominal Paracentesis 159
    Alan D. Miranda, M.D. and David R. Gerber, M.D.

Nutritional Immunomodulation in Surgical Patients 165
    Brian J. Daley, M.D. and Collin E. Braithwaite, M.D.

Physician Assistants: an Overview 177
    John F. Byrnes, Jr., PA-C

Physicians Assistants: a Cost-Efficient Solution for the Surgical
    Practice 183
    Linda A. Garry, PA-C and Debra L. Priore, PA-C

Future 2000 for Nurses 187
    Zane Robinson Wolf, PhD, RN

Contributors 195

Index 199

THE ROLE OF NUTRITION IN WOUND HEALING

Stanley J. Dudrick, M.D.

The University of Texas
Health Science Center at Houston
Hermann Hospital
Houston, Texas

It is generally recognized that a relationship exists between wound healing and the nutritional status of the patient, and it has been appreciated by surgeons for centuries that wound healing is impaired in patients with obvious malnutrition. Moreover, it was demonstrated more than 200 years ago that the wounds and poor wound healing associated with scurvy could be obviated or treated by the prevention or correction of a nutritional deficiency. Subsequently, knowledge of the mechanisms by which specific nutrient substrates and metabolites influence wound healing has ranged from virtually no data regarding some nutrients to a fairly well defined comprehension of the basic roles and kinetics of others. However, from a practical standpoint, clinicians in the industrialized nations such as the United States have the capability of rehabilitating depleted patients nutritionally by various means so that only rarely should nutritional deficiencies preclude major operations or give rise to serious wound complications. Indeed, ever since proteins were first discovered, it has been obvious clinically that normal protein metabolism and nutrition are essential for optimal wound healing.[1] Moreover, the wound healing process is better understood today to a large extent because of the extraordinary advances made in surgical nutrition in the second half of this century as a result of extensive investigations in basic and clinical nutrition. However, our knowledge concerning the wound healing mechanism in humans is still incomplete, primarily because of the difficulties inherent in designing and carrying out prospective, randomized, double-blind studies in this area either in patients or volunteer subjects. On the other hand, much valuable information has been accrued from wound healing experiments in animals and from empiric observations of human wound healing after surgery or trauma.

Early experimental studies demonstrated significantly impaired fibroplasia in the healing wounds of protein depleted rats[2] and dogs.[3] In the 1930's, Dr. I.S. Ravdin, at the University of Pennsylvania, focused his

Critical Issues in Surgery, Edited by A. C. Cernaianu et al.
Plenum Press, New York, 1995

laboratory efforts in the Harrison Department of Surgical Research on the nutritional problems of surgical patients.[4] He had been impressed, as had Jones and Eaton in Boston, with the edema that occurred in the intraperitoneal tissues of hypoproteinemic patients and thought that this might be the cause of the ileus and vomiting that occurred at times after major gastric operations in some patients.[5] He and his associates set out to reproduce these clinical conditions in a controlled comparable manner in dogs by feeding them a low protein diet, coupled with repeated plasmaphereses five or six times a week to lower serum protein levels to about 3 gm%. They showed clearly that gastric emptying was greatly retarded in all such animals that had also undergone gastroenterostomy and that the gastric emptying times returned to normal when the animals were returned to normal protein diets and regenerated their serum protein levels to normal. Subsequently, these investigators observed that their results were reproducible not only in animals with recent gastroenterostomies, but also in other animals who had undergone gastroenterostomy a year earlier, and even in some hypoproteinemic animals who had not undergone gastroenterostomy at all. Moreover, it was noted that the time required for a barium meal to traverse the small bowel from the pylorus to the cecum was similarly prolonged by, and correlated directly with, the degree of hypoproteinemia. In the course of these experiments, a number of wound disruptions occurred at the laparotomy sites, whereas previously, little or no difficulty with wound healing in any of the normoproteinemic animals studied in other various surgically oriented experiments had been encountered in these laboratories. Working with Thompson and Frank, Ravdin addressed this problem and showed that wound healing was significantly retarded in the hypoproteinemic animals and that the impaired wound healing was due to a great delay in fibroplasia.[6] Subsequently, several studies in animals suggested that protein depletion to the point of 20 percent weight loss interfered with repair of wounds.[7] These included the investigations of Dr. Jonathan E. Rhoads and associates, who demonstrated clearly a delay in laying down and calcifying callus in hypoproteinemic dogs who had undergone controlled Gigli saw fractures of the ulna.[8] In follow-up studies one year later, the same dogs healed identical fractures in the opposite ulna normally after their serum protein levels had been restored to normal. Since then, these observations have been confirmed by many investigators, and it has become apparent that a total body protein deficiency or an imbalance of specific amino acids has adverse effects on almost all aspects of wound healing, including neovascularization, lymphatic formation, fibroblast proliferation, collagen synthesis and wound remodeling. In the presence of prolonged protein deficiency or impaired liver function, local wound edema secondary to hypoalbuminemia may develop and further impair fibroplasia, especially of a healing intestinal or colonic anastomosis.[9]

At about the same time, Cannon and co-workers at the University of Chicago showed that resistance to infections was decreased by hypoproteinemia in rodents, and Wohl, at the Philadelphia General Hospital, corroborated these findings by demonstrating the delayed buildup of antibodies in hyproteinemic patients.[10,11] Brunschwig also showed a strong correlation between hypoproteinemia and infectious complications, including wound infection, and wound disruption after major operations.[12] Subsequently, Rhoads and Alexander confirmed these findings in a similar group of surgical patients at the Hospital of the University of Pennsylvania.[13] Meanwhile, the original work of Cuthbertson in Glasgow on the catabolic response to trauma in animals, which had been first reported in 1935, was becoming known to more investigators and clinicians around the world and was confirmed and extended to patients by Howard and his associates at Johns Hopkins.[14,15]

Although many similarities exist in the course of healing of connective tissue in different species of animals, it is not possible to transfer completely the information gained from animal experiments to clinical conditions in humans. For example, many differences exist between research animals and humans regarding the anatomy and the histologic appearance of the wound healing process. Relatively few wound healing studies have been performed in man for obvious reasons. However, it has been shown that the rate of healing of skin defects was faster in young patients than in old patients.[16] Baxter and associates studied specimens from patients given adrenocorticotrophic hormones and could demonstrate decreased rates of healing in some cases.[17] Wolfer and colleagues measured the decreased tensile strength of excised wounds in volunteers deficient in vitamin C.[18] The importance of zinc to wound healing has been demonstrated by Pories and co-workers by measuring the rate of decrease in the volume of the wound cavity after excision of pilonidal cysts.[19] Still others have quantitated the incorporation of specific amino acids such as radiolabeled cystine into the wound area, and Hunt and his associates have studied the role of oxygen content and oxygen consumption in wounds in human subjects.[20,21]

In other relevant areas of wound healing, particularly involving anastomoses of the gastrointestinal tract, practical problems associated with human studies are difficult to overcome. However, work has been done by Daly and co-workers to show that the healing and bursting strength of a rat colon anastomosis could be significantly affected by total serum protein levels, serum albumin concentrations and total circulating serum albumin.[9] An adverse effect on colon bursting strength was obtained whenever these indices were low, and the levels of serum total protein, serum albumin and total circulating serum albumin all correlated positively and linearly with the strength of an anastomosis of the colon or the small intestine in 5-7 days. Indeed, even the bursting strength of a segment of bowel one cm on either side of the anastomosis in a hypoproteinemic animal was less than the strength of an anastomotic site in a normoproteinemic animal studied concurrently. In follow-up of this work, Irvin studied the effects of enteral hyperalimentation on the healing of skin, abdominal and colonic wounds in malnourished rats.[22] The progressive weight loss induced in rats, starved of protein for seven weeks was accompanied by a significant reduction in the mechanical strength of sutured skin and abdominal wounds. A less pronounced but significant reduction in tensile strength of sutured colonic anastomoses was also demonstrated in these severely malnourished rats. When a group of malnourished rats were given oral supplements of amino acids and significantly higher daily caloric intake for one week before and one week after operation, nitrogen balance was achieved which was positive and consistently higher than in the untreated malnourished rats or the normal rats. Although the enteral amino acid therapy was associated with significant increases in the tensile strength and collagen content of the abdominal wounds, it had no measurable beneficial effects on the healing of skin wounds or colonic anastomoses. These results indicate that healing visceral and parietal tissues do not respond in a like manner to malnutrition or hyperalimentation therapy. Moreover, significant changes in wound healing occurred only in the presence of a severe degree of malnutrition when weight loss exceeded 1/3 of the normal body weight. The reasons for the different tissue responses to malnutrition are unknown, but results of previous studies of unwounded tissues by Harkness and co-workers and Caback and colleagues have also suggested that malnutrition has different effects on visceral and parietal tissues in mice and rats respectively.[23,24] It appears from their studies that visceral collagen is preserved to a much greater extent than is the collagen of skin or other parietal tissues such as the musculofascial layers of the abdominal wall.

In more recent work done at the University of Texas Medical School at Houston, a group of investigators has shown significant impairment of wound healing at the fracture site for the first time in a controlled study in malnourished humans.[25,26] Previous studies had demonstrated the impaired wound healing of a fracture when an animal was hypoproteinemic. However, this was the first work to show not only that the same was true for human patients, but that the impaired wound healing of the fracture could be accelerated when the patient was replenished nutritionally either with oral feeding, tube feeding, or total parenteral nutrition. These significant data really closed the circle that was opened by Cuthbertson when he first described the massive catabolism and protein loss associated with simple long bone fractures, initially in animals and later in humans.[14] Finally, the healing of test wounds in 108 patients was studied by Sandblom and colleagues, who reported that: 1) no differences in wound strength were noted between males and females; 2) no differences were noted when patients with malignancy were compared with comparable patients without malignant disorders; 3) patients with low serum albumin or low serum total proteins had significantly weaker wounds than patients with normal serum protein levels; and 4) patients over 80 years of age had poorer wound healing capabilities than those below age 70. This group also correlated their human data with their previous animal investigations and showed that in similar experiments, the wound strength in patients was identical with that in rats, slightly lower than that in rabbits, and significantly lower than that in pigs.[27]

In assessing patients with hypoproteinemia, which seems to be the single most important nutritional factor associated with impaired wound healing, the simplest and least sophisticated, but perhaps the most practical and available clinical parameter, for correlating wound healing with nutritional indices is the serum albumin concentration. Some clinicians have criticized the use of serum albumin concentration as a predictor of wound healing capability primarily because its level can vary significantly with changes in hydration and circulating blood volume. Additionally, serum albumin has a tendency to leak through the capillary walls into the interstitial spaces especially following major operative or accidental trauma or during sepsis, thus reducing its value as a marker of nutritional status under these conditions. Nonetheless, when hydration and blood volume considerations are taken into account in the same manner in which they must be factored when measuring serial hemoglobin and hematocrit levels to monitor blood loss or hematopoiesis, total serum protein and serum albumin levels correlate very well with the predicted ability of a patient to heal a wound, especially in the moderately severely and severely malnourished surgical patient.[28,29]

Clinical indices such as the appearance of the patient and findings on physical examination, degree and extent of recent weight loss, evidence of protein tissue loss, fluid retention, anemia, and low blood volume, total lymphocyte count or serum protein concentrations have been used as clinical guidelines in the evaluation of nutritional status and the prediction of the capability for, and rate of, wound healing in surgical patients. Increased sensitivity and correlation between protein status and wound healing can be obtained by measuring the serum concentration of transferrin, which has a shorter half-life than albumin. However, this is a much more expensive method by which to determine nutritional status. Even greater correlation can be shown between proteins and wound healing by measuring serum levels of pre-albumin and retinol binding protein, but at even greater expense.

Carbohydrates and fats have an important role in wound healing in that they can provide adequate energy and allow maximum sparing of endogenous and exogenous amino acid substrates for protein synthesis and collagen deposition by the fibroblasts. Little is known about the influence of fats on wound healing specifically although fatty acids are essential for transport across cell membranes. Attempts to assess the nutritional status of surgical patients in a more effective manner have recently been popularized originally by Blackburn and co-workers and subsequently by Mullen and co-workers.[28,30] The latter group of investigators have developed a prognostic nutritional index (PNI) based upon factors and constants derived from human experiments in which the serum albumin and transferrin levels, the triceps skin fold thickness, and delayed hypersensitivity manifested by skin testing were studied in a large number and wide variety of surgical patients. From these data a formula has been derived which can be used as an indicator either preoperatively or postoperatively for determining the patient's nutritional status and risk of postoperative complications including wound infection, impaired wound healing and wound disruption. In collaboration with the Department of Orthopedic Surgery at our own institution, nutritional assessment was carried out in 96 patients admitted for elective hip replacement. All patients were evaluated with a battery of 14 standard indices of nutritional assessment preoperatively. Based on our predetermined criteria for nutritional evaluation, 20 percent of this group were significantly malnourished, especially regarding their protein status. However, the protocol called for proceeding with whatever operation had been previously planned and without disrupting the original operative contract made between the patients and their orthopedic surgeons. At one month after operation, a 6 percent infection rate was noted in this group of patients which was about average for the nation. Subsequently, at one year following hip replacement, an 18 percent overall complication rate was noted in this group of patients, including delayed or indolent infection, wobbly prosthesis, and various other complications resulting in a failed operation as far as the orthopedic surgeon and patient were concerned. It is a highly relevant fact that both the 6 percent infection rate one month postoperatively and the 18 percent long-term complication rate one year postoperatively were derived entirely from the patients in the

20 percent group who were significantly malnourished as judged by our preoperative nutritional assessment criteria. Evaluation of these data resulted in the termination of the clinical study with the strong recommendation that all patients admitted to the hospital thereafter for elective hip replacement be assessed prior to admission, and should significant malnutrition be manifested, appropriate dietary consultation and measures for preoperative nutritional rehabilitation be instituted and implemented until the patient is replenished to normal nutritional status. Our experience to date indicates that normal nutritional status can be restored in about 10 days to three weeks of optimal oral or tube feeding in the average patient.[31]

We have developed a relatively simple, inexpensive and practical method for assessing nutritional status in our surgical patients. These criteria have proven useful in the management of a wide variety of complex surgical patients during the past 20 years and include: 1) an inadvertent, unintentional or unexplainable weight loss of 10 percent of body weight within the past one month; 2) a serum albumin level below 3.4 gm%; 3) an abnormally low total lymphocyte count (or   percent); and 4) evidence of impaired immunocompetence as determined by *in-vitro* studies and/or intradermal skin testing. If any one of these indices is abnormal, the patient is considered to be mildly malnourished. If any two indices are abnormal, the patient is considered to be moderately malnourished. If any three indices are abnormal, the patient is considered to be moderately severely malnourished. If all four indices are abnormal, the patient is considered to be severely malnourished. The incidence of postoperative complications correlates directly with the severity of the malnutrition, including impaired wound healing, wound infection and wound disruption. There is also a direct correlation between the level of malnutrition and mortality rate in addition to other forms of morbidity.

The effects of individual amino acids on healing have been shown to vary both quantitatively and qualitatively, and some investigators have shown that feeding the sulfur containing amino acids, methionine or cysteine, to protein deficient rats corrected the impaired healing to a significant degree by enhancing fibroblastic proliferation and collagen formation.[32-34] To date, the alterations in the metabolic priorities of specific amino acids following injury have not been well defined. Although changes in the plasma concentrations of various amino acids and their metabolites have been described, knowledge of the mechanisms by which these changes affect the metabolism of the individual amino acids at the cellular and organ levels is lacking. All biological amino acids are essential for optimal wound healing and tissue repair. However, following injury, the requirements for certain amino acids which are ordinarily synthesized at rates adequate for maintenance of homeostasis may increase, requiring augmented dietary intake. This is manifested by the fact that when supplementary arginine is administered, it can accelerate the healing of wounds in rats fed a normal rat chow diet.[1,35]

Decreased hydroxyproline content of the wound has been demonstrated in malnourished patients, but can be reversed by intravenous nutrition.[36] Since the advent of total parenteral nutrition techniques, many surgeons have noted healing of previously indolent wounds and even of fistulas of the type which formerly would not have been expected to heal, and the conviction that protein-calorie nutrition is important to wound healing and tissue repair is growing.[7] However, from a clinical standpoint, many wounds heal remarkably well despite severe protein-calorie malnutrition. This phenomenon has been described by the concept of a so-called protected wound module in which adequate healing can sometime proceed despite systemic malnutrition.[37]

Prior to the development and clinical application of intravenous hyperalimentation or total parenteral nutrition, the management of internal and external fistulas of the gastrointestinal tract was accompanied by high morbidity and high mortality rates.[38-40] Virtually all patients with such complications suffered from some degree of nutritional depletion which was aggravated further by the adverse effects of the fistula. Although the nutritional deficits were obvious, a successful feeding technique for correcting them was not available. The level of the fistula within the gastrointestinal tract was the primary variable that either prohibited or permitted some form of successful enteral feeding via the available bowel. Fistulas in the distal portions of the gastrointestinal tract (distal ileum or colon) generally responded favorably to alimentary tract feeding because a greater mucosal surface is available for absorption of ingested nutrients proximal to the fistula, whereas fistulas in the upper gastrointestinal tract (duodenum or proximal jejunum) more often than not were associated with high incidences of complications, therapeutic failure, and death. For many years prompt operation or re-operation was recommended for all upper gastrointestinal tract (high output) fistulas, and operative mortality was high. In those patients who survived operation, the incidence of recurrent fistula as a result of anastomotic failure was also high. The use of the technique of total parenteral nutrition and bowel rest has obviated the necessity for urgent or emergency operation for fistula closure, has allowed the nutritional status of the patient to be restored to normal or near normal, and has yielded much more satisfactory results than in the past. Subsequently, the development of elemental diets and other specially formulated enteral diets for oral or tube feeding have accomplished similar results in patients in whom a reasonable amount of small bowel was available for efficient absorption.

In our initial combined series of more than 100 consecutive patients with enterocutaneous and enteroenteral fistulas, an overall 70.5 percent rate of spontaneous closure was achieved. The overall mortality rate in this group of patients was 6.45 percent, compared with mortality rates of 40 percent and 65 percent in two different previously published large series of patients.[38,39] Operation was required to close the fistulas in 21.8 percent of the patients, and the mortality rate was 6.7 percent in this group. The remaining 7.7 percent of the fistulas never closed, and all of these patients died. Of particular significance were the closure rates of the enterocutaneous fistulas of the upper gastrointestinal tract. Fifty percent of the gastric fistulas, 100 percent of the duodenal fistulas, and 87.5 percent of the jejunal fistulas closed spontaneously. These results undoubtedly reflect the fact that total parenteral nutrition significantly reduces the secretory activity of the organs of the upper alimentary tract while concomitantly providing adequate nutrient substrates for restoration of nutritional status.[41] Similar results have been achieved in the nonoperative management of pancreatic fistulas for the same reasons.[42] Subsequently, several studies have validated these data, and it appears logical to assume that the provision of adequate nutritional support by parenteral and/or enteral means has revolutionized the management of patients with fistulas of the alimentary canal as manifested not only by the highest rate of spontaneous closure ever achieved, but more importantly by the striking decline in morbidity and mortality rates among patients with these rather special wounds and healing problems.

Considering the rapidity with which events occur at the molecular level during the healing of a wound, it is not surprising that a variety of metabolic and nutritional factors can influence wound healing in dramatic ways. Moreover, the nature and magnitude of the injury are often so great that a wide variety of physiological, metabolic and nutritional disorders can result which themselves can influence wound healing. Furthermore, the underlying nutritional condition of the patient prior to the injury or operation can have a profound influence on healing mechanisms. Additionally, wounds can be quite complex, involving several different tissues or organs, each with its own distinctive anatomical and physiological characteristics, and healing can be complicated by microbial contamination, devitalized tissue, foreign bodies, and compromised blood supply. Finally, it requires emphasis that problems related to wound healing and wound infection are intricately related, and that metabolic and nutritional factors affect resistance to infection in the same manner as they affect wound healing.[1]

Disorders of carbohydrate and fat metabolism have both indirect and direct effects on wound healing. Indirect effects occur as a result of excessive oxidation of amino acids for caloric needs when inadequate amounts of carbohydrate and fat are available. Progressive amino acid and protein depletion follow, leading to secondary adverse effects on wound healing. When glucose is not present in adequate amounts, the direct effect of this deficiency is that the energy requirements of cells including leukocytes and fibroblasts are not met. As a result, wound healing is impaired and resistance to infection is decreased. If the period of metabolic and physiological derangement is prolonged, caloric requirements should be supplied to seriously injured patients as unsaturated fatty acids in twice the minimum recommended intake for healthy individuals. Although there is evidence suggesting that requirements for essential fatty acids are increased after severe burns, no studies have been reported on the effects of specific fatty acid deficiencies on wound healing.[1]

Following injury, especially extensive third degree burns, vitamin C metabolism and flux change dramatically so, that despite a large intake of ascorbic acid and a low urinary excretion of ascorbic acid, the plasma ascorbic acid level can be low, and tissue saturation tests can show marked depletion. The mechanisms underlying these disturbances have not been established. However, it has been suggested that the rate of ascorbic acid metabolism may be increased and that ascorbic acid accumulates in the areas of the injured tissues. Since vitamin C is not stored to any great extent in the body, seriously injured patients may develop ascorbic acid deficiency rapidly unless ascorbic acid is supplemented aggressively in the dietary regimen. However, no evidence exists that wound healing can be accelerated by administering more vitamin C than is required to maintain normal tissue levels. Clinical scurvy is very rarely seen today, but its biochemical sequelae have been well studied and include inhibition of collagen synthesis and subsequent cross-linking.[37]

Very little data exist regarding the specific effects of the B-complex vitamins on wound healing. On the other hand, serious deficiencies of some of these vitamins can interfere with healing because the B vitamins serve as co-factors in a wide variety of enzyme systems, and their absence can cause disturbances in protein, carbohydrate and fat metabolism. Moreover, deficiencies of the B-complex vitamins can lead to major adverse effects on resistance to infection. Ordinary daily doses appear to be sufficient to satisfy the needs of wound repair.

Vitamin A accelerates the healing of skin incisions and the formation of granulation tissue and stimulates repair of steroid retarded wounds. Since vitamin A is stored in the liver, it is unlikely that a deficiency will develop following uncomplicated elective surgical operations. However, it is recommended that supplemental vitamin A be given to all patients with severe injury, especially major burns, beginning as soon as possible since the need for vitamin A is accentuated under hypermetabolic conditions regardless of the patient's previous nutritional status. Recommendations vary from 10,000 IU/day for most patients to 25,000-50,000 IU/day for major burn patients.

There is no clear evidence of a specific role for vitamin E in wound healing or for an alteration in vitamin E metabolism or requirement following injury. Indeed, in rats, it has been shown in some experiments that vitamin E actually suppresses wound inflammation and collagen synthesis and antagonizes vitamin A.

It has been suggested that vitamin D is essential to soft tissue repair, but the evidence is not convincing. However, vitamin D is essential to normal calcium metabolism, and its deficiency can lead to osteomalacia and poor fracture healing. There are no known increased losses of vitamin D following routine surgical procedures, and ordinary daily dietary requirements are sufficient for most surgical patients and trauma patients.

In clinical conditions including severe injury, infection, and disorders of the gastrointestinal tract, zinc deficiency can occur, and the patient will likely have wound healing problems when total body zinc levels are low. This can be prevented or corrected by administering supplemental zinc in the diet. However, giving zinc to a patient who is not zinc deficient does not improve or accelerate wound healing above normal and actually may be detrimental if excessive amounts are given.

Many specific nutritional requirements of wound healing and tissue repair remain poorly defined. The individual nutritional substrates whose deficits have been shown to have an adverse effect on wound healing have been presented. It is clear that a wide variety of metabolic and nutritional factors influence wound healing and that their effects on the patients' reparative systems are complex, additive, and sometimes synergistic. Total parenteral nutrition can be a potent tool in providing the nutrient requirements not only for basal maintenance, but for the accentuated needs following injury or major surgical procedures. However, its use is accompanied by the implied responsibility that the intravenous nutrient solutions are formulated and administered in a manner to insure the provision of all substrates in quantities and ratios to correct or prevent any deficiencies. Until the time when all of the contributions of individual nutrients and nutrient substrates to optimal wound healing can be defined, surgeons and other clinicians are advised to maximize efforts to provide a balanced nutritional regimen by whatever technique possible to achieve optimal wound healing and tissue repair in seriously ill or injured patients.[43]

Finally, it should be re-emphasized that the wound healing process is so complicated by the presence of microorganisms, immunologic status, the extent of devitalized tissue and efficiency of debridement, the characteristics of the materials used and the techniques used for approximating wounds and other tissues, etc., that it is very difficult to determine the relative importance of each of the individual contributors or components essential to an optimally healing wound. Thus, the difficulties encountered in standardizing wounds, suturing techniques, wound management and extraneous factors render it almost impossible in a clinical setting to obtain highly significant wound healing data in response to the manipulation of individual nutrient moieties. However, it is important to remember that at the tissue level, wound healing fundamentally is a biochemical process; that nutrition support actually is clinical biochemistry; and that an obvious relationship between the two exists. Food must be thought of as anything of biological value that is ingested into the gastrointestinal tract; diet as that combination of foods which are ingested over a specific period of time; but nutrition as the individual molecular nutrient substrates that are delivered at any time to the specific cells and across their membranes in support of their vital biochemical activities. Thus, nutrition really occurs at the cell membrane and in the cell, and only when the quality and quantity of the nutritional support is equal or superior to the technical, mechanical and other aspects of wound healing, will the surgeon's goal of optimal wound healing be realized.

REFERENCES

1. Levenson SM, Seifter E: Dysnutrition, wound healing and resistance to infection. Clin Plastic Surg 1977;4:375.
2. Howes EL, Briggs H, Shea R, Harvey SC: Effects of complete and partial starvation on the rate of fibroplasia in the healing wound. Arch Surg 1933;27:846.
3. Rhoads JE, Fliegelman MT, Ponzer LM: The mechanism of delayed wound healing in the presence of hypoproteinemia. JAMA 1972;118:21.
4. Jones CM and Eaton FG: Postoperative nutritional edema. Arch Surg 1933;27:159.
5. Mecray PM, Barden RP, Ravdin IS: Nutritional edema: Its effect on gastric emptying time before and after gastric operations. Surgery 1937;1:53.
6. Thompson WB, Ravdin IS, Frank IL: Effect of hypoproteinemia on wound disruption. Arch Surg 1938;35:500.
7. Hunt, TK: Nutritional requirements of repair. In Ballinger WF, et al. (eds). Manual of Surgical Nutrition by the Committee on Pre- and Postoperative Care, American College of Surgeons, Philadelphia, WB Saunders, 1975.
8. Rhoads JE, Kasinskas W: Influence of hypoproteinemia on the formation of callus in experimental fracture. Surgery 1942;11:38.
9. Daly JM, Vars HM, Dudrick SJ: Effects of protein depletion on strength of colonic anastomosis. Surg Gynecol Obstet 1972;134:15.
10. Cannon PR, Wissler RW, Woolride RL, Beditt EP: Relationship of protein deficiency to surgical infection. Ann Surg 1944;120:514.
11. Wohl MD, Reinholdt JG, Rose SB: Antibody response in patients with hypoproteinemia. Arch Int Med 1949;83:402.
12. Brunschwig A, Clark DE, Corbin N: Symposium on Abdominal Surgery: Postoperative nitrogen loss and studies on parenteral nitrogen nutrition by means of casein digest. Ann Surg 1942;115:1091.

13. Rhoads JE, Alexander CE: Nutritional problems of surgical patients. Ann NY Acad Sci 1955;63:268.
14. Cuthbertson DP: Further observations on the disturbance of metabolism caused by injury, with particular reference to the dietary requirements of fracture cases. Brit J Surg 1935;23:505.
15. Howard JE, Parson W, Slen KE, Eisenberg H, Reidt V: Studies on fracture convalescence. I. Nitrogen metabolism after fracture and skeletal operations in healthy males. Bull Johns Hopkins Hosp 1944;75:156.
16. DuNouy PL: Cicatrization of wounds: Mathematical expression of the curve representing cicatrization. J Exp Med 1916;24:451.
17. Baxter H, Schiller C, Whiteside J: Influence of ACTH on wound healing in man. Plast Reconstr Surg 1951;7:85.
18. Wolfer JA, Farmer CJ, Carroll WW, Manshardt DO: An experimental study in wound healing in vitamin C depleted human subjects. Surg Gynecol Obstet 1947;84:1.
19. Pories WJ, Henzel JH, Rob CG, Strain WH: Acceleration of wound healing in man with zinc sulfate given by mouth. Lancet 1967;1:121.
20. Haley HB, Williamson MB: The healing of human wounds. In vivo studies. Surg Forum 1957;8:62.
21. Hunt TK, Ninikoski J, Zederfeldt B: Role of oxygen in repair processes. Acta Chir Scand 1972;138:109.
22. Irvin TT: Effects of malnutrition and hyperalimentation on wound healing. Surg Gynecol Obstet 1978;146:33.
23. Harkness M, Harkness RD, James DW. The effect of a protein-free diet on the collagen content of mice. J Physiol 1958;144:307.
24. Caback V, Dickerson JWT and Widdowson EM. Response of young rats to deprivation of protein or of calories. Br J Nutr 1963;17:601.
25. Heard CW, Jr, Griffith RB, Smith TK, Daly JM, Dudrick SJ: Improved fracture healing in severely traumatized rats treated with total parenteral nutrition. J Parent Ent Nutr 1982;6:331.
26. Jensen JE, Jensen TG, Smith TK, Johnston DA, Dudrick SJ: Nutrition in orthopaedic surgery. J Bone Joint Surg 1982;64A:1263.
27. Lindstedt E, Sandblom P: Wound healing in man: Tensile strength of healing wounds in some patient groups. Ann Surg 1975;181:843.
28. Buzby GP, Mullen JL, Matthews DC, Hobbs CL, Rosato EF: Prognostic nutritional index in gastrointestinal surgery. Am J Surg 1980;139:160.
29. Casey J, Flinn WR, Yao JST, Fahey V, Pawlowski J, Bergan JJ: Correlation of immune and nutritional status with wound complications in patients undergoing vascular operations. Surgery 1983;93:822.
30. Blackburn GL, Bistrian BR, Maini BS, Schlamm HT, Smith MF: Nutritional and metabolic assessment of the hospitalized patient. J Parent Ent Nutr 1977;1:11.
31. Jensen JE, Smith TK, Jensen TG, Dudrick SJ, Butler JE, Johnston DA: Nutritional assessment of orthopaedic patients undergoing total hip replacement surgery. In Klein EA (ed): The Hip, Volume 9, St. Louis, Mosby Times Mirror, 1982.
32. Localio SA, Morgan ME, Hinton JW: The biological chemistry of wound healing. The effect of methionine on the healing of wounds in protein-depleted animals. Surg Gynecol Obstet 1948;86:582.
33. Williamson MB, Fromm HJ: The incorporation of sulfur amino acids into proteins of regenerating wound tissue. J Biol Chem 1955;212:705.
34. Edwards LC, Dunphy JE: Methionine in wound healing during protein starvation. In Williamson MD (ed): The Healing of Wounds, London, McGraw-Hill, 1957.
35. Barbul A, Fiskel RS, Shimazu S, et al: Intravenous hyperalimentation with high arginine levels improves wound healing and immune function. J Surg Res 1985;30:328.
36. Haydock DA, Hill GL: Improved wound healing response in surgical patients receiving intravenous nutrition. Br J Surg 1987;74:320.
37. Coit DG: Care of the surgical wound. In Wilmore DW, et al. (eds) Care of the Surgical Patient by the Committee on Pre- and Postoperative Care, American College of Surgeons, New York, Scientific American, Inc., 1988.
38. Edmunds H, Jr, Williams GM, Welch CE: External fistulas arising from the gastro-intestinal tract. Ann Surg 1960;152:445.

39. Sheldon GF, Gardiner BN, Way LW, Dunphy JE: Management of gastro-intestinal fistulas. Surg Gynecol Obstet 1971;133:385.
40. Chapman R, Foran R, Dunphy JE: Management of intestinal fistulas. Am J Surg 1964;108:157.
41. MacFadyen BV, Jr, Dudrick SJ, Ruberg RL: Management of gastrointestinal fistulas with parenteral hyperalimentation. Surgery 1973;74:100.
42. Dudrick SJ, Wilmore DW, Steiger E, Mackie JA, Fitts WT, Jr: Spontaneous closure of traumatic pancreatoduodenal fistulas with total intravenous nutrition. J Trauma 1970;10:542.
43. Ruberg RL: Role of nutrition in wound healing. Surg Clin North Am 1984;64:705.

CHRONIC WOUNDS: GROWTH FACTORS AND COMPREHENSIVE SURGICAL CARE

David R. Knighton, M.D.

Institute for Reparative Medicine
St. Louis Park, Minnesota

Nonhealing chronic cutaneous ulcers are a significant clinical, social, and healthcare problem. Patients with chronic nonhealing wounds have many different clinical problems which result in the formation of chronic cutaneous ulcers. These include: peripheral vascular arterial and venous disease, autonomic and sensory neuropathy, impaired host defense against infection, and delayed wound repair. To effectively treat these patients and heal the ulcers all the complicating factors must be addressed. In this chapter, we will discuss the surgical care of these patients and the use of topically applied platelet releasates which contain growth factors in combination with a comprehensive treatment algorithm.

NORMAL WOUND REPAIR

The regulation of wound repair is a complex and constantly changing field. A superficial description of the overall process is summarized below.

Initiation of Repair

When trauma creates a wound space, the traumatic tissue disruption exposes plasma to connective tissue proteins activating factor XII. Activated factor XII, in turn, activates the clotting, kinin, complement, and plasmin cascades. The clotting cascade produces thrombin and fibrin. Thrombin stimulates platelets to release α granules which contain growth factors, matrix molecules and protease inhibitors needed for repair. Fibrin produces the first matrix which fills the wound space. The kinin cascade produces bradykinin which causes microvascular vasodilation at the wound edge to increase circulation in the patent capillaries. Complement activation produces C5a which brings neutrophils and monocytes into the newly formed wound space. Plasmin is produced which degrades the fibrin, starting the

Critical Issues in Surgery, Edited by A. C. Cernaianu et al.
Plenum Press, New York, 1995

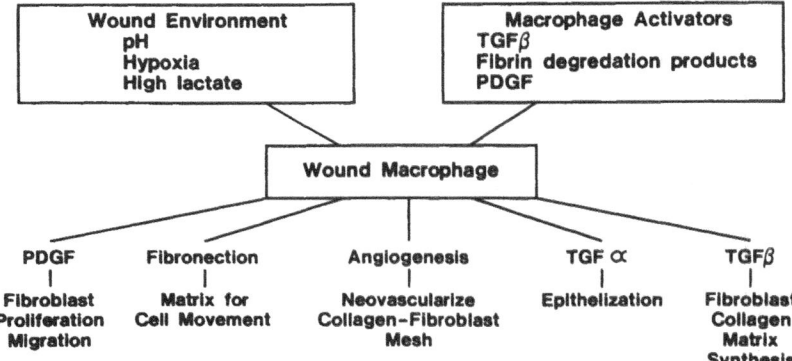

Figure 1. Schematic diagram depicting the ability of the wound macrophage to regulate the wound healing response. In response to environmental and biochemical signals, the macrophage produces various mediators of tissue repair

remodeling process and releasing fibrin degradation products which are also chemoattractants for macrophages and probably *activate* them as well.[1]

Cellular Production of Locally Acting Growth Factors

The release of platelet α granules into the wound space is thought to be one of the principle sources of growth factors which triggers connective tissue formation. Platelet derived growth factor (PDGF), transforming growth factor-β (TGF-β), platelet factor 4 (PF4), β-thromboglobulin (BTG), fibronectin and thrombospondin, plasminogen activator inhibitor and other factors are released. Neutrophils and monocytes are the first cells recruited from the host which populate the wound space. They control bacterial contamination of the wound and clear cellular debris. Monocytes mature into wound macrophages which produce growth factors. Macrophages continue to release PDGF, TGF-β, transforming growth factor-α (TGF-α), and lactate throughout wound repair (Figure 1).[2] The combination of PDGF, TGF-β, and potentially other platelet and macrophage released growth factors produce a vascularized connective tissue matrix which fills the wound space. PDGF also stimulates wound contraction. Epidermal growth factor (EGF), TGF-α and potentially TGF-β, stimulate epidermal cells to migrate and divide to cover the granulation tissue. Platelets could play a continuing role in growth factor production throughout repair due to leakage of platelets through the loose junctions in newly formed capillaries..

Termination of Repair

There are at least two schools of thought about how healing ends. As the wound heals, the size of the wound space decreases as it is filled with a vascularized connective tissue matrix. One school contends that tissue growing from the wound edge completely fills the wound space and this returns the microenvironment of the space to that of *normal* vascularized connective tissue. This return may help signal the wound to stop repair since the oxygen tension will be high enough to shut off macrophage lactate and angiogenesis factor production.[3] In addition, new microvasculature produced by angiogenesis factor is initially very leaky. Plasma, red cells and platelets continually leak through the loose junctions releasing serum mediators and platelet growth factors. When the wound space is filled, no further angiogenesis occurs and the microvasculature matures to form tight junctions and a basement membrane. This stops the leak of plasma and cells, and may shut off an important source of growth factors. The result of this return of the wound space to normal connective tissue conditions tends to inhibit release of angiogenesis factors and perhaps other stimulators of repair. A second potential mechanism involves active inhibition of growth factor activity by the process of epithelization and production of inhibitors of angiogenesis, fibroplasia, and epithelization.

GROWTH FACTORS AND REPAIR

The cellular activities associated with wound repair appear to be regulated by locally acting growth factors. These biomolecules, usually small polypeptides, stimulate and possibly control cell proliferation, movement and biosynthetic activity. They can act as paracrine (produced by one cell type to act on another in the local area) or autocrine (produced by a cell acting on itself) factors. This is a rapidly changing field, and new growth factors with potential roles in wound repair are continually being isolated and characterized. The general categories of growth factors with specific examples of their roles in wound healing are discussed.

Locally acting growth factors can be grouped into three large categories: 1) mitogens which signal cells to proliferate, 2) chemoattractants which stimulate cellular migration, and 3) transforming growth factors which alter the phenotypic state of the cell.

Mitogens can be divided into *competence* and *progression* factors. In order to divide, cells must be stimulated to progress from the resting state (G0) to a state of readiness to replicate DNA and divide (G1). So called *competence* factors appear to stimulate cells to make this transformation. Once cells enter G1, progression through the division cycle seems to require the presence of progression factors.[4] Platelet derived growth factor (PDGF) and epidermal growth factor (EGF) are examples of competence factors. Known progression factors include insulin-like growth factor (IGF-1) and the other somatomedins. These progression factors circulate in plasma and are readily available to cells stimulated to enter G1 by the competence factors. There is also evidence that they are secreted by fibroblasts in wounds and in this way act as autocrine factors.

Chemoattractants can be divided into chemotactic factors and chemokinetic factors. Chemotactic factors work through cell surface receptors which on reaching one side of a cell in higher concentrations than the other cause the target cell to move in a given direction. Examples of chemotactic factors are C5a which is a chemoattractant for neutrophils and PDGF which is a chemoattractant for fibroblasts.[5,6] Chemokinetic factors increase the rate of cell migration, but not in a directional manner.[7] An example of chemokinesis is the effect of albumin on neutrophil migration and fibroblast growth factor on endothelial cells.[8] Many growth factors act as both mitogens and chemoattractants depending on concentration and target cell.

The most studied transforming growth factor is transforming growth factor β (TGFβ). TGFβ is reported to have a variety of activities, dependent on the cell type affected and the microenviroment in which it is acting.[9] In certain concentrations, it inhibits fibroblast division and stimulates increased production of matrix molecules (collagen and glycosaminoglycans). It also induces the production of PDGF in certain cells. Transforming growth factor α (TGFa) shares considerable homology with EGF, binds to the same receptor, and evokes many of the same responses as EGF.[10,11]

The biochemical and biological activities of the certain growth factors presently thought to play a role in the regulation of wound repair are briefly summarized below.

Platelet Derived Growth Factor (PDGF)

PDGF is a 30,000-32,000 Dalton glycoprotein made up of two disulfide linked subunits.[12] Originally discovered in platelets, this competence factor has been found in monocytes, smooth muscle cells, endothelial cells, and various transformed cells.[13-16] It binds to high affinity receptor sites, is active in the picomolar range, and is a potent mitogen for most mesenchymally derived connective tissue cells.[17] As mentioned above, it is both a chemotactic molecule and a competence factor.

Epidermal growth factor (EGF)

EGF is a 6,000 Dalton protein made up of a single chain of 53 amino acids.[18] It binds to high affinity receptors and is found in platelets, salivary glands, duodenal glands, and urine.[19-22] It is a competence factor for many epithelial and mesenchymal cells and stimulates epidermal regeneration after partial thickness injuries.[23]

Transforming Growth Factor β (TGFβ)

TGFβ is a 25,000 Dalton protein made up of two chains. It is secreted from the cell as a high molecular weight precursor which is cleaved at low pH.[24,25] It is acid and heat stable and binds to high affinity receptors on the target cell. TGFβ is found in many cells including platelets, macrophages, and lymphocytes.[9] It inhibits cellular proliferation, is a monocyte chemoattractant and stimulates macrophages to produce many monokines, and stimulates collagen and fibronectin production from fibroblasts and keratinocytes.[26-30] *In vitro* it has been shown to stimulate endothelial cells to form tube-like structures.[31]

Angiogenesis Factors

Angiogenesis is the process of new capillary formation. It is poorly understood in terms of the actual growth factor regulation since the potential list of *angiogenesis factors* is long and continues to grow. Angiogenesis involves at least 5 cellular events: endothelial cell protease production, endothelial cell migration, endothelial cell proliferation, endothelial cell tube formation and extracellular matrix synthesis. Ultrastructural studies on capillary proliferation demonstrate that capillary endothelial cell migration with enzyme production are the first activities seen, followed by endothelial cell proliferation.[32,33]

NONHEALING WOUNDS

There are many reasons why the healing process is interrupted resulting in a non-healing cutaneous ulcer. Essentially, there are five main reasons why wounds don't heal: 1) infection, 2) ischemia, 3) repeated trauma, 4) metabolic abnormalities, and 5) medications. Many patients have all five problems resulting in a complex interaction which must be completely understood and treated before wound repair can occur. Others have only one problem, which when corrected, often results in prompt repair.

INFECTION

All cutaneous wounds are exposed to bacteria. During the process of successful wound repair, the original bacterial inoculum is controlled by the neutrophil/monocyte based, host defense system. When the patient is unable to effectively control and eliminate the bacterial inoculum, the normal process of wound repair is either delayed or stopped. If the bacterial proliferation goes unchecked, the resulting infectious necrosis of the peri-wound tissue can significantly increase the total wound burden.

ISCHEMIA/HYPOPERFUSION

The process of wound repair requires energy. Any pathologic process which interrupts delivery of oxygen and nutrients to the cells involved in normal repair can result in delayed healing. Decreased oxygen and blood flow can result from a deficiency in any portion of the oxygen/blood flow pathway which ends in oxygen delivery to the cell. Common areas of impairment include inadequate oxygenation due to chronic lung disease and congestive heart failure, deficient delivery due to arterial stenosis or obstruction, impaired cellular delivery due to increased tissue edema from venous disorders, or decreased capillary perfusion due to increased tissue pressure, and deficient cellular nutrient/oxygen utilization due to enzyme deficiency or pharmalogic manipulation. Restoring adequate blood flow and oxygen/nutrient delivery is critical if healing is to occur.

REPEATED TRAUMA

The process of wound repair requires an orderly sequence of cellular events. If during the healing process repeated injury continually destroys the new tissue, a non-healing wound can result. The repeated injury could be due to repeated excessive tissue pressure which interrupts blood flow resulting in tissue ischemia and necrosis. Repeated injury resulting in continual breakdown of the protective epithelial barrier can lead to persistent invasive infection. Uncontrolled inflammation due to a connective tissue disorder or foreign body can create a cellular micro-environment which prevents connective tissue formation and wound repair.

MEDICATIONS

Administration of topical or systemic medication often affect or impair a critical event in wound repair. Many of the topical antimicrobials are toxic to connective tissue cells. Their use may decrease the alterial bacterial of the wound, but significantly delay the repair process. Medications which modulate the inflammatory process, such as steroids and non-steroidal anti-inflammatory agents significantly delay repair by impairing the necessary early signals which start wound healing. Chemotherapeutic agents used to treat cancer and some connective tissue disorders affect wound repair by killing the rapidly dividing cells necessary for prompt wound repair.

TREATMENT OF CHRONIC CUTANEOUS ULCERS

The treatment of chronic cutaneous ulcers requires a systematic approach to address the five principal causes on non healing. These include adequate control of blood sugar, correction of macrovascular arterial occlusions, control of local factors which affect tissue oxygen transport such as edema and infection, aggressive tissue debridement to decrease the infectious burden and determine the total wound burden, adequate antibiotic therapy to control tissue infection, unweighting the wound area to minimize local trauma, and tailoring the topical and systemic medications to minimize the effects on wound repair. Attention to these tenets of wound care is essential. In addition, the use of newer technologies such as topical application of growth factors holds promise to not only accelerate but alter the character of wound healing in the diabetic.

To determine the effect of a particular intervention, such as growth factor administration, on wound repair requires careful monitoring of the state of ischemia, infection, trauma, and patient compliance, along with the wound repair endpoints, including infection control, granulation tissue formation, and epithelization. At present, the most completely studied and used growth factors in chronic wounds are the naturally occurring mix of growth factors from the α-granule of the platelet. This mixture of growth factors, protease inhibitors, and matrix molecules is called Platelet Derived Wound Healing Formula (PDWHF).

PDWHF is an autologous solution made from the patient's own blood. Blood is withdrawn from the patient, the platelets are extracted from the blood and the growth factors are released from the platelets by the addition of thrombin. The product of platelet α granule release including growth factors are resuspended in a solution which allows them to stay active.

PDWHF contains at least five locally acting growth factors fromα-granulates: platelet-derived growth factor (PDGF),[34] β thromboglobulin, platelet-derived epidermal growth factor (PDEGF),[35] transforming growth factor-β (TGF-β),[36] and platelet factor 4 (PF4).[34]

CLINICAL TRIALS

Four clinical trials have documented the effectiveness of this comprehensive approach to the chronic nonhealing wound.

1. Prospectively randomized double-blind placebo-controlled trial of PDWHF.[37]
2. A multicenter, prospectively randomized, double-blind trial.
3. Two limb salvage studies. One on patients recommended for amputation[38] and a second study where a panel of experts on amputation were case reviews to determine the severity of the wound and predict whether amputation was necessary.

DOUBLE-BLIND, RANDOMIZED, CROSSOVER, PLACEBO-CONTROLLED TRIALS

To test the independent efficacy of PDWHF, a double-blind, crossover, placebo-controlled trial was performed.[37] A total of 32 patients were randomized into treatment and control groups. All patients received standard wound care as described above. The placebo was the platelet buffer combined with microcrystalline collagen without plateletα granule release products. Patients randomized to the control group had their blood drawn and the PDWHF stored for use after the crossover period. Both groups were treated for a total of 8 weeks and then the placebo patients were crossed over to the positive arm of the study, treatment with PDWHF.

When the patient populations in each group were analyzed and wounds graded using the wound grading system, the two groups were matched except for the area measurement. Patients randomized to the control group had a higher area measure than control due to 2 patients with very large wounds.

A total of 13 patients finished the positive arm. Eleven patients finished the control arm. In the positive arm, 17 out of 21 total wounds achieved 100 percent epithelization in an average of 8.6 weeks. In the placebo group of 11 patients, 2 out of 13 wounds (15 percent) healed during the initial 8 weeks of placebo treatment, and 11 of 13 wounds (85 percent) failed to heal in 8 weeks and were crossed over to the positive group. After crossover, all 11 nonhealed wounds achieved 100 percent epithelization in an average of 7.1 weeks. When analyzed statistically, there is a high degree ($p < 0.0002$) of significance between the two groups.

The second prospectively randomized, double-blind, placebo-controlled trial was a multicenter study. Ninety-seven patients were randomized into one of four treatment groups: three different doses of homologous thrombin induced platelet releasate or the placebo. Sixteen patients were removed from the study because they did not meet protocol criteria and eleven more were removed for patient noncompliance. The study period lasted for 20 weeks or until the wounds were completely healed. Efficacy was determined by evaluating percent total healing and the rate of area and volume reduction in 70 diabetic patients. The results of the study showed that each group receiving the platelet releasate stimulated greater healing than the placebo group. The best results were achieved in the 0.01 dilution group. Eighty-percent of the wounds healed vs 29 percent of the placebo group (p=0.01), volume reduction was 94.9 percent in the 0.01 dilution vs 82.7 percent in the placebo group (p=0.005). No differences or trends were found in the adverse event profiles between active product and placebo groups.[39]

LIMB SALVAGE STUDIES

Many of the patients referred to the clinic have threatened limbs due to ischemic nonhealing wounds. We retrospectively studied 24 of these patients to determine if treatment in the clinic under defined protocols with the use of PDWHF resulted in limb salvage.[38]

Patients were studied if they had ischemic nonhealing extremity ulcers that required amputation according to their referring physician. Recommended amputations at the transmetatarsal level (TMA) or higher were included. Minor amputations of the toes were not included. Success was defined as 100 percent epithelialization of the wound, progressive epithelial maturation, and the ability to tolerate limited weight bearing.

The patients ranged in age from 28 to 80 years, with 9 patients (38 percent) 65 years or older. The primary diagnosis was diabetic mellitus in 21 patients (88 percent), atherosclerotic peripheral vascular disease in 2 patients (8 percent), and rheumatoid arthritis in 1 patient (4 percent). All patients over the age of 65 had diabetes mellitus.

Eleven patients had 15 prior amputations, 7 patients had 10 prior vascular procedures, and 6 of these 7 patients had vascular reconstructions in the limb that was now threatened.

The referring physician recommended below-the-knee amputation (BKA) in 18 patients, TMA in 5 patients, and a ray amputation in 1 patient (this patient was included because he needed a BKA on our evaluation).

The patients had 26 ulcers. The mean duration of conventional unsuccessful therapy was 26 weeks, with a range of 3 to 43 weeks.

As far as other factors are concerned, 46 percent (11 of 24) of the patients smoked and 21 percent (5 of 25) were on steroids (4 for renal transplantation and 1 for severe rheumatoid arthritis).

Arteriograms were performed in 13 of 24 patients (54 percent), 11 of 24 patients (45 percent) underwent vascular reconstruction, and 20 of 24 patients (83 percent) had operative wound debridement before beginning PDWHF therapy.

The patients were followed for an average of 15 months, with a range of 7 to 29 months. Follow-up data was obtained from their last clinic visit or phone conversation.

Of the 24 patients, 4 required amputation. Two patients' wounds did not heal. One required an above-the-knee amputation, the other a below-the-knee amputation. The other two patients' wounds were healing. One had a clotted vascular bypass resulting in amputation and the other developed necrotizing soft tissue infection from walking on a plantar surface ulcer; both required below-the-knee amputations.

In all, 19 of 24 patients (79 percent) healed 21 of 26 wounds. Two patients' wounds recurred after healing; one of these patients' wounds healed a second time by the end of the study. Two patients were still healing at the end of the study, leaving a total of 18 of 24 patients (75 percent) healed with 20 of 26 wounds (77 percent) healed. Most important, 17 of 18 patients who healed are ambulatory, with one healed patient unable to ambulate because of a previous stroke. The 2 patients who were still healing are on restricted ambulation. Of the 4 amputees, 2 ambulate on prostheses and 2 are nonambulatory.

A second study on amputation prevention involved an independent review panel composed of an orthopedic surgeon, a vascular surgeon, and an endocrinologist. They conducted a blinded retrospective review of 71 diabetic patients with 124 wounds on 81 limbs. Based on their expertise, the review panel classified the wounds severity and identified the limb's risk for amputation. Their judgement was compared to the actual outcome.

The review panel predicted 65 (80 percent) of the limbs would be salvaged and 16 (20 percent) would be amputated. The actual outcome was that 75 (93 percent) of the limbs were salvaged and 6 (7 percent) were amputated ($p<0.005$). This study demonstrated that the combination of aggressive revascularization and debridement, infection control, and unweighting of plantar ulcers, along with the use of PDWHF, was very effective in amputation prevention.

CONCLUSIONS

The care of chronic cutaneous ulcers is a complex therapeutic process where meticulous attention must be paid to all the contributing processes which cause the ulcer. When this is accomplished, the rate and success of wound repair can be accelerated and increased through the proper use of adjunctive agents such as growth factors.

REFERENCES

1. Dvorak HF, Kaplan AP, Clark RAF: Potential functions of the clotting system in wound repair. The Molecular and Cellular Biology of Wound Repair. In: Clark RAF, Henson PM (eds), Plenum Press, New York, NY, 1988:57-85.
2. Rappolee DA, Mark D, Banda MJ, Werb Z: Wound macrophages express TGF-alpha and other growth factors in vivo: Analysis by mRNA phenotyping. Science 1989;241:708-712.
3. Knighton DR, Hunt TK, Scheuenstuhl H, Halliday BJ, Werb Z, Banda MJ: Oxygen tension regulates the expression of angiogenesis factor by macrophages. Science 1983;221:1283-1285.
4. Deuel TF: Polypeptide growth factors: Roles in normal and abnormal cell growth. Ann Rev Cell Biol 1987;3:443-492.
5. Snyderman R, Philips J, Mergenhagen SE: Polymorphonuclear leukocyte chemotactic activity in rabbit serum and guinea pig serum treated with immune complexes: Evidence for C5a as the major chemotactic factor. Infect Immun 1970;1:521-525.
6. Seppa H, Grotendorst G, Seppa S, Schiffmann E, Martin GR: Platelet-derived growth factor is chemotactic for fibroblasts. J Cell Biol 1982;92:584-588.

7. Wilkinson PC: Chemotaxis and chemokinesis: Confusion about definitions. J Immunol Methods 1988;110:143-144.

8. Wilkinson PC, Allan RB: Assay systems for measuring leukocyte locomotion: An overview. Leukocyte Chemotaxis: Methods, Physiology and Clinical Implications. In: Gallin JI, Quie PG (eds). Raven Press, New York, NY, 1978:1-24.

9. Sporn MB, Roberts AB, Wakefield LM, de Crombrugghe B: Some recent advances in the chemistry and biology of transforming growth factor-beta. J Cell Biol 1987;105:1039-1045.

10. Massague J: Epidermal growth factor-like transforming growth factor: Isolation, chemical characterization, and potentiation by other transforming factors from feline sarcoma virus transformed rat cells. J Biol Chem 1983;258:13606-13620.

11. Derynck R, Roberts AB, Winkler ME, Chen EY, Gueddel DV: Human transforming growth factor alpha: Precursor structure and expression in E. coli. Cell 1984;38:287-297.

12. Raines EW, Ross R: Platelet-derived growth factor I. High yield purification and evidence for multiple forms. J Biol Chem 1982;257:5154-5160.

13. Martinet Y, Bitterman PB, Mornex JF, Grotendorst GR, Martin GR, Crystal RG: Activated human monocytes express the c-sis protocogene and release a mediator showing PDGF-like activity. Nature 1986;319:158-160.

14. Walker LN, Bowen-Pope DF, Ross R, Reidy MA: Production of PDGF-like molecules by cultured arterial smooth muscle cells accompanies proliferation after arterial injury. Pro Natl Acad Sci USA 1986;83:7311-7315.

15. DiCorleto PE, Bowen-Pope DF: Cultured endothelial cells produce a platelet-derived growth factor-like protein. Pro Natl Acad Sci USA 1983;80:1919-1923.

16. Deuel TF, Huang JS: Platelet-derived growth factor: Structure, function and roles in normal and transformed cells. J Clin Invest 1984;74:669-676.

17. Ross R, Raines EW, Bowen-Pope DF: The biology of platelet derived growth factor. Cell 1986;45:155-169.

18. Taylor JM, Mitchell WM, Cohen S: Epidermal growth factor: Physical and chemical properties. J Biol Chem 1972;247:5928-5934.

19. Oka Y, Orth DN: Human plasma epidermal growth factor/betaurogastrone is associated with blood platelets. J Clin Invest 1983;72:249-259.

20. Kasselberg AG, Orth DN, Gray ME, Stahlman MT: Immunocytochemical localization of human epidermal growth factor/urogastrone in several human tissues. J Histochem Cytochem 1985;33:315-322.

21. Olsen PS, Poulsen SS, Kirkegaard P: Adrenergic effects on secretion of epidermal growth factor from Brunner's glands. Gut 1985;26:920-927.

22. Gregory H: Isolation and structure of urogastrone and its relationship to epidermal growth factor. Nature 1975;257:325-327.

23. Brown GL, Nanney LB, Griffen J, Cramer AB, Yancey JM, Curtsinger LJ, Holtzin L, Schulte GS, Jurkiewicz MJ, Lynch JB: Enhancement of wound healing by topical treatment with epidermal growth factor. N Engl J Med 1989;321:76-80.

24. Pircher R, Jullien P, Lawrence DA: Beta-transforming growth factor is stored in human blood platelets as a latent high molecular weight complex. Biochem Biophys Res Commun 1986;136:30-37.

25. Lawrence DA, Pircher R, Jullien P: Conversion of a high molecular weight latent beta-TGFb from chicken embryo fibroblasts into a low molecular weight active beta-TGFb under acidic conditions. Biochem Biophys Res Commun 1985;133:1026-1034.

26. Moses HL, Tucker RF, Leof EB, Coffey RJ, Halper J, Shipley GD: Type beta transforming growth factor is a growth stimulator and a growth inhibitor. Cancer Cells (Cold Spring Harbor) 1985;3:65-71.

27. Wahl SM, Hunt DA, Wakefield LM, McCartney-Francis N, Wahl LM, Roberts AB, Sporn MB: Transforming growth factor type beta induces monocyte chemotaxis and growth factor production. Proc Natl Acad Sci USA 1987;84:5788-5792.

28. Wiseman DM, Polverini PJ, Kamp DW, Leibovich SJ: Transforming growth factor-beta (TGF-B) is chemotactic for human monocytes and induces their expression of angiogenic activity. Biochem Biophys Res Commun 1988;157:793-800.

29. Ignotz R, Massague J: Transforming growth factor-beta stimulates the expression of fibronectin and collagen and their incorporation into the extracellular matrix. J Biol Chem 1986;261:4337.
30. Wikner NE, Persichitte KA, Baskin JB, Nielsen LD, Clark RAF: Transforming growth factor-beta stimulates the expression of fibronectin by human keratinocytes. J Invest Dermatol 1988;91:207-212.
31. Madri JA, Pratt BM, Tucher AM: Phenotypic modulation of endothelial cells by transforming growth factor beta depends upon the composition and organization of the extracellular matrix. J Cell Biol 1989;106:1375-1384.
32. Folkman J: Angiogenesis. Biology of Endothelial Cells. Jaffe EA (ed). Martinus Nijhoff Publishers, Boston, MA, 1984:412.
33. Knighton DR, Phillips GD, Fiegel VD: Wound healing angiogenesis: Indirect stimulation by basic fibroblast growth factor. J. Trauma 1990;30(12):S134-S144.
34. Kaplan KL, Broekman MJ, Chernoff A, Lesznik GR, Drillings M: Platelet alpha-granule proteins: Studies on release and subcellular localization. Blood 1979;53:604-618.
35. Oka Y, Orth DN: Human plasma epidermal growth factor/betaurogastrone is associated with blood platelets. J Clin Invest 1983;72:249-259.
36. Assoian RK, Sporn MB: Type-beta transforming growth factor in human platelets: release during platelet degranulation and action on vascular smooth muscle cells. J Cell Biol 1986;102:1217-1223.
37. Knighton DR, Ciresi K, Fiegel VD, Schumerth S, Butler E, Cerra F: Stimulation of repair in chronic, nonhealing, cutaneous ulcers using platelet-derived wound healing formula. Surg Gynecol Obstet 1990;170:56-60.
38. Knighton DR, Fylling CP, Fiegel VD, Cerra FB: Amputation prevention in an independently reviewed at-risk diabetic population using a comprehensive protocol and platelet-derived wound healing formula. Am J Surg 1990;160(5):466-471.
39. Holloway GA, Steed DL, DeMarco MJ, Masumoto T, Moosa HH, Webster MW, Bunt TJ, Polansky M: A randomized, controlled, multicenter, dose response trial of activated platelet supernatent, topical CT-102 in chronic, nonhealing, diabetic wounds. Wounds 1993;5(4):198-206.

WOUND HEALING AND INFECTION

Donald E. Fry, M.D.

University of New Mexico School of Medicine
Albuquerque, New Mexico

Inflammation is a ubiquitous tissue response that has many specific elements. Inflammation has many important tissue-level functions that represent components of host defense. The inflammatory response represents the primary biological method for tissue hemostasis following injury. It serves the critical role for the localization, containment, and irradication of potential microbial pathogens which contaminate tissue. Furthermore, inflammation is the initial phase responsible for wound healing.

Ordinarily, these three functions of inflammation function at separate and independent times. The inflammatory response serves its hemostatic function within the first 10-15 minutes following injury. Coagulation proteins, platelets, and local vasoconstriction are rapidly activated to arrest local blood loss. The precipitation of fibrin at the exposed wound surface becomes a biological defense against secondary contamination that may subsequently assault the open injury. Local responses of increased vascular permeability mediated by inflammatory proteins from mast cells create tissue edema which facilitates the delivery of important plasma proteins. Tissue edema may also provide the aqueous channels for the prompt delivery of neutrophils into the areas to eliminate microbes, foreign bodies, and devitalized tissue. At 12-24 hrs, macrophage cells begin to migrate into the area and become important in modulation of neutrophil phagocytic activity, but also to promote the orchestration of the wound healing process. The fibrin matrix which is precipitated about the injury site becomes the tissue-level scaffolding upon which fibroblasts will synthesize collagen. When all goes well, the collagen synthesis process will be a significant process by the fourth-to-fifth day following injury. Fibrin is systemically replaced by collagen as wound tensile strength is enhanced over the subsequent weeks following the injury. In wound healing, inflammation functions to provide the lattice-work for collagen repair and to recruit the cellular elements responsible for collagen production.

The premise of this presentation will be that each phase of the inflammatory response must achieve its biological end-point before the next phase of the process can be initiated. Importantly, when clinical infection occurs within the wound, the active products produced by phagocyte-patho-

Critical Issues in Surgery, Edited by A. C. Cernaianu et al.
Plenum Press, New York, 1995

gen interaction become destructive to the subsequent processes of wound healing. Infection delays wound healing. Furthermore, when systemic infection or the systemic inflammatory response syndrome is activated, it is contended that systemic re-prioritization leads to a delay in wound healing even in areas that are remote from the primary process.

BIOLOGY OF WOUND INFECTION

With penetration of the epidermis, bacterial contaminants gain access to the soft tissues and become potential pathogens to the host. The number of bacterial contaminants is highly variable and depends upon the mechanism and circumstances of injury. Traumatic injuries generally have large bacterial counts and are also affected by adjuvant factors in the wound. These adjuvant factors include hemoglobin, foreign bodies, dead tissue, and dead space that each have an amplifying effect upon the virulence of the bacterial contaminants.

The bacterial contaminants themselves, exposed collagen from the injury, and extravasation of red blood cells become stimuli to initiate the inflammatory response. While activation of the coagulation cascade has purpose for hemostasis, it also becomes the initial non-specific element of host defense. Coagulation protein precipitation creates a matrix about would-be pathogens to prevent tissue invasion and provide a containment defense. The fibrin matrix becomes a primary barrier to potential secondary contamination from microbes that are not part of the initial injury.

Following acute injury and hemostasis, mast cells release inflammatory proteins which result in vasodilation and increased vascular permeability. Tissue edema results from the suffusion of plasma proteins into the injured area. Additional fibrin is precipitated and complement cleavage products are released which combined with mast cell proteins and prostaglandin metabolic products now become chemoattractants, or biological beacons, to attract phagocytic cells into the area of injury.

The diffusion of chemoattractants from the epicenter of injury provides direction for phagocytic cells. Margination of neutrophils to vascular endothelium is followed by diapedesis towards the chemical focus. Free microbes and foreign debris stimulates the process of phagocytosis, which is followed by intracellular killing and digestion. Enzymatic digestion of the fibrin matrix surface by proteases from the neutrophil appears to facilitate neutrophil access to bacteria that are entrapped. The number of neutrophils and the vigor of the phagocytic process is governed initially by the number of bacteria, the degree of tissue destruction, and the magnitude of complement activation.

Beginning at 12-24 hours after injury, the macrophage cell now migrates into the area. If the magnitude of contamination and tissue injury is small, then pro-collagen synthesis cytokine signals are released and the process of mesenchymal cell differentiation is triggered by transforming growth factor-β, platelet-derived growth factor, and probably other known and undefined cytokine signals.[1] However, severe contamination with bacteria accompanied by dead tissue may rather stimulate the proinflammatory cytokine response including tumor necrosis factor (TNF) and the various interleukin cytokines. TNF serves the role of a paracrine message and fully activates neutrophils into a frenzied state of phagocytic activity.[2] Vigorous extracellular release of hydrophilic, proteolytic, and lysosomal enzymes result in extracellular digestion of adjacent tissue. Rapid digestion of the fibrin matrix occurs. The natural end-point of this phagocytic pathogen interaction is the formation of pus. Thus, pus constitutes partially digested host proteins, fibrin proteins, dead leukocytes, and bacteria with varying degrees of viability. Drainage of pus to the exterior reduces the pro-inflammatory stimulus which hopefully leads to the macrophage reprioritization to cytokine production for the mode of pro-collagen synthesis.

In the surgical wound, events are similar to that of a traumatic wound. However, certain differences are important and underscore the potential adverse effects of fibrin deposition. The surgical incision develops a fibrin interface against the external environment. Surgical trauma, retraction of the wound edges, stretching, and abrasion of the wound during the operation means that fibrin continues to be precipitated such that the thickness of the matrix continues to increase during the procedure. Contamination continues from the environment and from endogenous sources. Thus, the microscopic assessment of the fibrin layer would reflect the levels of contamination during the operation. In a colon resection for example, the fibrin layers closest to the subcutaneous tissue itself would be relatively free of bacteria since this layer would correlate with the opening of the abdomen and reflect the *clean* component of the procedure. The more superficial layers of the fibrin matrix would reflect the period of the procedure when the colon was opened and the anastomosis was performed. Much higher bacterial concentrations would be expected at this level of the fibrin matrix. At the completion of the procedure, the wound closure represents the apposition of two contaminated fibrin surfaces to one another, a biological event not anticipated by the evolutionary forces of wound healing. The edema process continues during and following wound closure and results in a perimeter of increased hydrostatic pressure about the incision interface. This results in the primarily closed wound being relatively ischemic due to this incisional "halo" of increased tissue pressure.

Wound infection becomes the result when the number of bacterial contaminants exceed a critical threshold, usually perceived to be 10^5 organisms/gram of wound tissue.[3] The actual number may be less because of the amplification effects of adjuvant effects. Thus, Elek identified that a 100-fold reduction in the number of contaminants would still cause experimental wound infection if a foreign body (eg. silk suture material) were present in the wound.[4]

The natural history of the inflammatory response, as the first phase of both host defense and wound healing, and of wound infection helps explain the value and the limitations of antibiotics in the prevention of surgical wound infection. Miles et al demonstrated that systemic antibiotics could prevent dermal infection if the antibiotic was present in the tissue at the time of contamination.[5] Antibiotics given greater than three hours after contamination had no impact upon the natural history of the disease. Polk and Lopez-Mayor demonstrated the clinical usefulness of preventive antibiotics in patients undergoing elective gastrointestinal surgery.[6] Stone et al. noted that antibiotics started in the postoperative period had no benefit in the prevention of wound infections.[7] Stone also demonstrated that preoperative antibiotics alone with a postoperative placebo for five days was as effective as the same preoperative antibiotic and five postoperative days of the drug.[8] Antibiotics must be present in the wound fluid at the time of contamination if prevention is to be achieved.[9]

Because the fibrin matrix is virtually impervious to systemically administered antibiotics given after the fibrinogen-to-fibrin transformation, fibrin is hypothesized to be a major explanation for the ineffectiveness of post-contamination preventive antibiotics. For antibiotics to be effective in prevention, the drug must be present in the serum and entrapped within the fibrin matrix at the time of bacterial contamination. Furthermore, the ischemic perimeter about the closed surgical wound means that systemic drug given after wound closure poorly penetrates the wound interface and certainly would be poorly effective in penetrating the would fibrin matrix. Thus, the biological mechanism to entrap bacteria and prevent tissue invasion, results in retardation of phagocytic access to the fibrin-encased pathogen and also compromises the use of post-contamination antimicrobials in the prevention of infection.

INFECTION AND WOUND HEALING

The traditional phases of wound healing in the infection include inflammation, collagen synthesis, epithelialization, remodeling, and contraction of the wound. The processes when unaccompanied by infection occur in a systematic fashion. Inflammatory events characterize the first 72 hours after injury. Collagen synthesis and epithelialization begin as the inflammatory phase subsides. Remodeling and contraction may continue for a year thereafter.

Infection in the wound disrupts the entire progression of events.[10] The fibrin matrix which becomes the scaffolding for collagen deposition is destroyed and digested by both the bacterial pathogen and by the host response to infection. Bacterial proteases normally released to facilitate environmental digestion to provide microbial nutrients readily digest the lattice-work of fibrin. More important than the bacteria themselves is the host response to the microbes. The up-regulation of neutrophil activation by the effects of TNF, complement cleavage products, and even endotoxin directly through the CD14 receptor mechanism[11] results in frenzied fibrin digestion via acid hydrolases, lysosomal enzymes, and reactive oxygen intermediates of neutrophil origin.

The active infection process results in the extension of the acute inflammatory process into adjacent and previously unaffected wound tissues. This results in more activation of mast cells, more activation of the complement cascade, and the generation of more chemoattractants. Large concentrations of chemoattractants from the epicenter of the active infection draw more neutrophils to the area. The environment that is rich in chemoattractants, bacterial cell products, and pro-inflammatory macrophage cytokines may lead to full activation of the neutrophil cells within the vascular compartment at the time of margination, but prior to migration into the soft tissue. The intravascular release of potent digestive enzymes and reactive oxygen intermediates leads to microcirculatory thrombosis. Hence, wound ischemia develops in a progressive fashion and results in additional tissue necrosis.

The consequence of wound ischemia and the competition of bacterial pathogens with host phagocytic cells for the available oxygen in the microenvironment is profound wound hypoxia. Wound hypoxia compromises the ability of host phagocytic cells to kill bacterial pathogens through oxygen-dependent pathways.[12] Wound hypoxia suppresses macrophage-mediated fibroblast proliferation and appears to secondarily impair the wound healing process.[13]

The entire microenvironment becomes a battleground of proinflammatory host enzymes against bacterial invaders. The reparative *peace* process of wound repair becomes fully subservient to the tissue destructive focus of pro-inflammatory host responses. Resolution of the infection and cessation of the sustained inflammatory state is necessary before wound healing can proceed.

Considerable evidence would support the position that a yen-yang relationship exists in the wound between the pro-inflammatory forces and the pro-collagen synthesis forces. Macrophage cells appear to be primarily responsible for the production of both the pro-inflammatory TNF,[14] and the pro-collagen synthesis cytokine transforming growth factor-β (TGF-β).[15] It is unclear whether a given macrophage within the wound produces both cytokines at the same time and that the quantitative production of one over another results in the net biological effect. Production of one cytokine may result in the down-regulation of the other. Other important growth factors, such as platelet-derived growth factor,[16] must also have their effects neutralized by the pro-inflammatory effects of TNF.

Nevertheless, acute wound infection leaves the macrophage to orchestrate the inflammatory response through TNF and other interleukin cytokines, but the absence of TGF-β effects means that mesenchymal precursor cells destined to become fibroblasts are not so stimulated until the pro-inflammatory event has subsided. Indeed, evidence indicates that topical TNF retards wound healing while antibodies to mouse-TNF given to animals after acute wounding actually accelerates wound healing.[17] Furthermore, topical TGF-β in acutely created wounds appears to abrogate acute pro-inflammatory events and accelerates wound healing.[18] Thus, while events within the wound probably dictate the active synthetic pathways of pro-TNF or pro-TGF-β, the interaction of these two macrophage products at the interface areas between infected and non-infected portions of the same wound probably assumes biological significance.

The process of epithelialization of the wound is clearly affected by active infection. Locally destructive digestive neutrophil products probably provide a logical explanation for the failure of epithelialization and contraction. Recent data identified bacterial exotoxins as interfering with epithelialization and contraction and suggests that bacterial products themselves may be responsible for these observations.[19] Another plausible explanation would again focus upon the proinflammatory stimulus that exotoxin would have upon the host phagocytic and inflammatory response as being the final common mediator for inhibition of wound healing. Similar effects have been seen when active gram negative infection of the wound is created without apparent exotoxin production.[20] From this author's perspective, it seems more likely that destructive products derived from neutrophils are of greatest significance to altered wound healing, than are bacteria-derived products.

An intriguing paradigm in the saga of infection-related impairment of wound healing is the impact of remote infections. Some data would support the position that a distant infection such as pneumonia might delay the healing of an abdominal incision that was not itself infected. While TNF and TGF-β appear to be primarily paracrine signals that promote the biological sequelae of wound healing within a local tissue domain, the potential endocrine scope of these and other pro-inflammatory and pro-collagen synthesis signals becomes an interesting source of speculation. Does a disseminated signal from a septic source inhibit collagen synthesis at a remote wound site? While current evidence to support this potential scenario is lacking, this area should be an important and exciting focus for future investigation.

REFERENCES

1. McGrath MH: Peptide growth factors and wound healing. Clin Plast Surg 1990;17:421-432.
2. Klebanoff SJ, Vedes MA, Harlan JM, et al: Stimulation of neutrophils by tumor necrosis factor. J Immunol 1986;136:42204225.
3. Robson MC, Krizek TJ, Heggers JP: Biology of Surgical Infections. In Current Problems in Surgery. Year Book Medical Publishers, Chicago,IL, March 1973.
4. Elek SD, Conen PE: The virulence of staphylococcus pyogenes for man: a study of the problem of the wound. Br J Exper Pathol 1957;38:573.
5. Miles AA, Miles EM, Burke JF: The value and duration of defense reactions of the skin to the primary lodgment of bacteria. Brit J Exper Pathol 1957;38:79-96.
6. Polk HC Jr, Lopez-Mayor JF: Postoperative wound infection: A prospective study of determinant factors and prevention. Surgery 1969;66:97-103.
7. Stone HH, Hooper CA, Kolb LD, et al: Antibiotic prophylaxis in gastric, biliary, and colonic surgery. Ann Surg 1976;184:443-452.
8. Stone HH, Haney BB, Kolb LD, et al: Prophylactic and preventive antibiotic therapy: Timing, duration, and economics. Ann Surg 1979;189:691-699.
9. Fry DE, Pitcher DE: Antibiotic pharmacokinetics in surgery. Arch Surg 1990;125:1490-1492.
10. Robson MC, Stenberq BD, Heggers JP: Wound healing alterations caused by infection. Clin Plast Surg 1990;17:485-492.
11. Wright SD, Ramos RA, Tobias PS, et al: CD14 serves as the cellular receptor for complexes of lipopolysaccharide with lipopolysaccharide binding protein. Science 1991;249:1431-1433.
12. Knighton DR, Halliday B, Hunt TK: Oxygen as an antibiotic: a comparison of the effects of inspired oxygen concentration and antibiotic administration on in vivo bacterial clearance. Arch Surg 1986;121:191-195.
13. Bankey P, Fiegel V, Singh R, et al: Hypoxia and endotoxin induce macrophage-mediated suppression of fibroblast proliferation. J Trauma 1989;29:972-980.
14. Beutler B, Cerami: Cachectin: More than a tumor necrosis factor. N Engl J Med 1987;316:379-385.
15. Sporn MB, Roberts AB, Wakefield LM, de Crombrugghe B: Some recent advances in the chemistry and biology of transforming growth factor-beta. J Cell Biol 1987;105:1039-1045.
16. Mustoe TA, Purdy J, Gramates P, et al: Reversal of impaired wound healing in irradiated rats by platelet-derived growth factorBB. Am J Surg 1989;158:345-350.
17. Regan MC, Kirk SJ, Hurson M, et al: Tumor necrosis factor-alpha inhibits in vivo collagen synthesis. Surgery 1993;113:173177.
18. Cromack DT, Porras-Reyes B, Purdy JA, et al: Acceleration of tissue repair by transforming growth factor-beta-1: Identification of in vivo mechanism of action with radiotherapy-induced specific healing deficits. Surgery 1993;113:36-42.

19. Heggers JP, Haydon S, Ko F, et al: Pseudomonas aeruginosa exotoxin A: its role in retardation of wound healing: the 1992 Lindberg Award. J Burn Care Rehab 1992;13:512-518.

20. Stenberg BD, Phillips LG, Hokanson JA, et al: The effect of bFGF on the inhibition of contraction of the wound caused by bacterial contamination. Surg Forum 1989;40:629-631.

THE *PLUG* REPAIR FOR RECURRENT INGUINAL HERNIAS

Alex G. Shulman, M.D.

Lichtenstein Hernia Institute
Los Angeles, California

Most surgeons view the prospect of repairing a recurrent inguinal hernia with well justified anxiety. The prospect of undertaking such an operation is bad enough if it is a patient referred to the operating surgeon. It is even worse if this is one's own recurrence. Concerns usually relate to the finding of scarred tissues, often resulting in totally unrecognizable anatomy. When dissected, the tissues bleed easily and the results are generally poor and uncertain. In addition, the remaining blood supply to and from the testis may be compromised during the current repair and there is always a possibility of a malpractice lawsuit.

The outcome of standard methods of repairing recurrent hernias is unacceptable. After the first recurrent hernia repair, one can expect a 25 to 30 percent failure rate. Following the second, the rate increases to 50 percent. The repair of a third or fourth recurrence almost always results in 100 percent failure rate.

Why do such poor results occur with standard recurrent hernia repairs? We feel very strongly that the dissection of the entire floor of the inguinal canal to try to create a new stronger floor is unnecessary. Usually a large hernia replaces a small one. The newly created leaves of the floor of the inguinal canal must be resewn using old scarred tissues which are poorly vascularized and much more rigid than in the prior procedure. In addition, one should consider that the repair has already failed under better circumstances. To expect a high degree of success under such conditions is illogical.

What then is the answer? For approximately 80 percent of recurrent hernias, there is a rather simple solution which is based on almost 2,000 patients referred to us in the past 25 years. One should consider the nature of the defects found in recurrent inguinal hernias. They are located primarily lateral to the pubic bone and at the internal orifice of the inguinal ligament. Such defects are solitary in approximately 95 percent, since any pressure against the hernial opening simply enlarges it but is not likely to create a second defect. The diameter of such a defect is 3.5 cm or less in approxi-

Critical Issues in Surgery, Edited by A. C. Cernaianu et al.
Plenum Press, New York, 1995

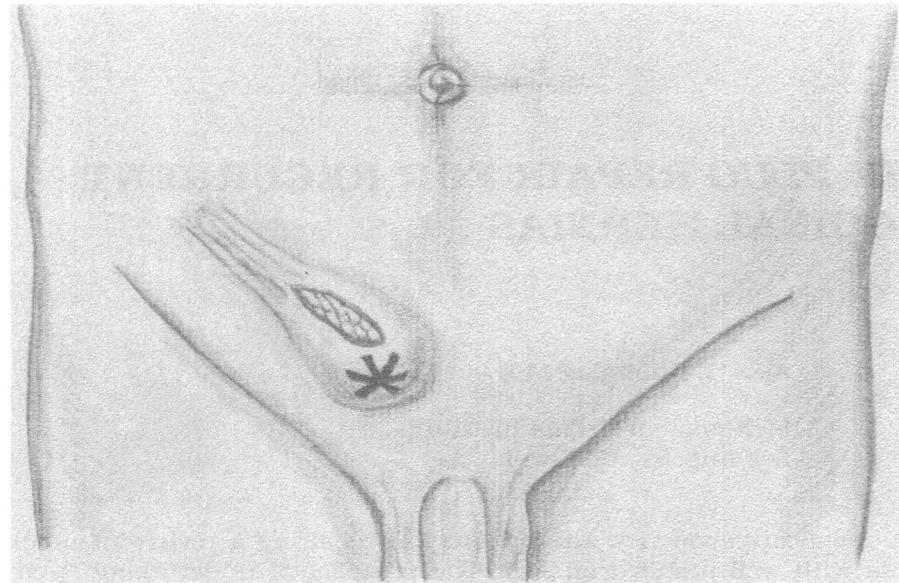

Figure 1. Skin mark to aid in locating the hernia sac.

mately 80 percent of such cases.[1,2] Based on these facts, the great majority of recurrent hernias may respond to treatment by the insertion of a mesh plug to close the defect (Plan A).

SURGICAL TECHNIQUE

The critical point of this technique is the location of the hernial sac. We recommend placement of a heavy ink mark on the skin to show the exact location of the bulge (Figure 1).

The hernia should be carefully checked when the patient is both in the standing and in the supine position, since the sac frequently falls away and disappears when the patient lies flat on his back. However, when the patient is under general or spinal anesthesia, there is no help to be expected from the patient in trying to locate the hernial sac. For that reason, recurrent hernias are treated under local anesthetic and the patient knows beforehand he is expected to cooperate by coughing and straining on command. Since these patients have already experienced a previously failed repair, most patients are extremely cooperative at this next operation. Under exceptional circumstances, such as a large recurrence in a very obese patient, a paravertebral anesthetic block may be needed. For such patients with an obvious bulge, it is not necessary to have the patient's cooperation in finding the hernia. Under local anesthesia, a short incision, usually under 4 cm, is begun and is placed adjacent to the skin mark but generally within a portion of the old scar (Figure 1). The subcutaneous tissues contain the spermatic cord, which is always completely flattened out and frequently lying over the hernial sac. It is sometimes difficult to find the sac, but the

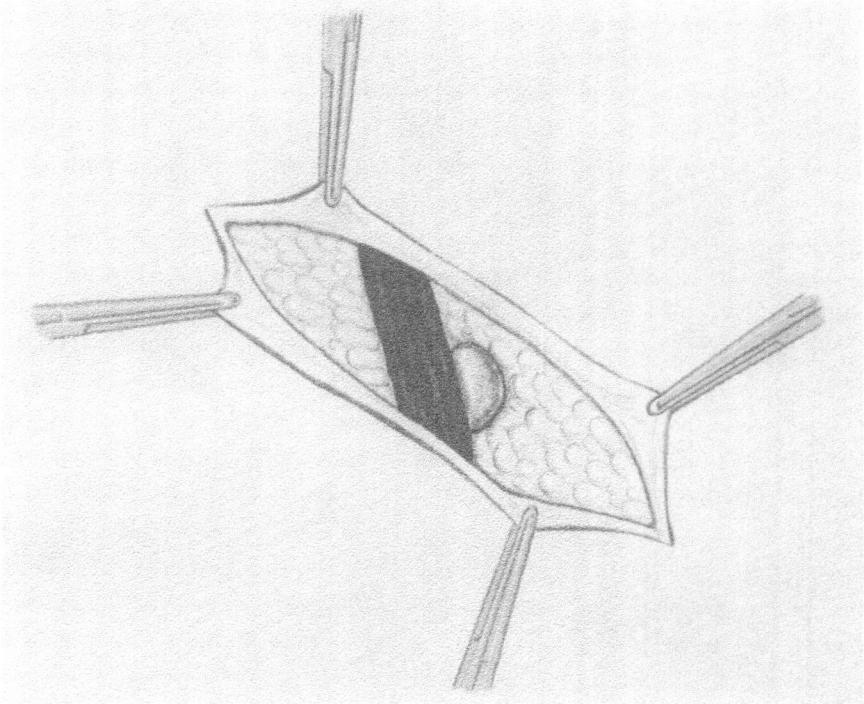

Figure 2. Sac frequently under flattened spermatic cord.

patient's frequent coughing and straining will help the surgeon to locate it. Once it is found (Figure 2), it is dissected towards it as depth hugging the sac and avoiding any traumatic retraction of the spermatic cord if possible (Figure 3).

As the sac is further dissected, usually the first opening found can be mistaken for the hernial defect, however, this is probably the old external ring. It is necessary to dissect the sac all the way down to the peritoneal level. Here, a firm, often scarred ring is identified. It is usually made up of tissues which cannot be named with any certainty. The sac is cleared from the margins of the defect and returned to the peritoneal cavity without ligation. Following this, a finger insertion into the defect examines the remainder of the floor of the inguinal canal for a possible second defect, which rarely exists. A Marlex® mesh plug is now made in the following manner.

It is necessary to begin with a sheet of mesh which will create a plug that is 2 cm wide and 20 to 30 to 40 cm or even longer in order to create the full plug that is demanded. By folding the 8 x 16 cm sheet into four lengthwise, so that it is four layers thick, one can create a combined strip 2 cm wide and 64 cm long. If it is found to be too small, which is rarely the case, more mesh can be added. If it is too large, it can be trimmed to fit. The plug is constructed by winding the mesh around a Kelly clamp placed transversely at one end of the mesh until the appropriate size is obtained.

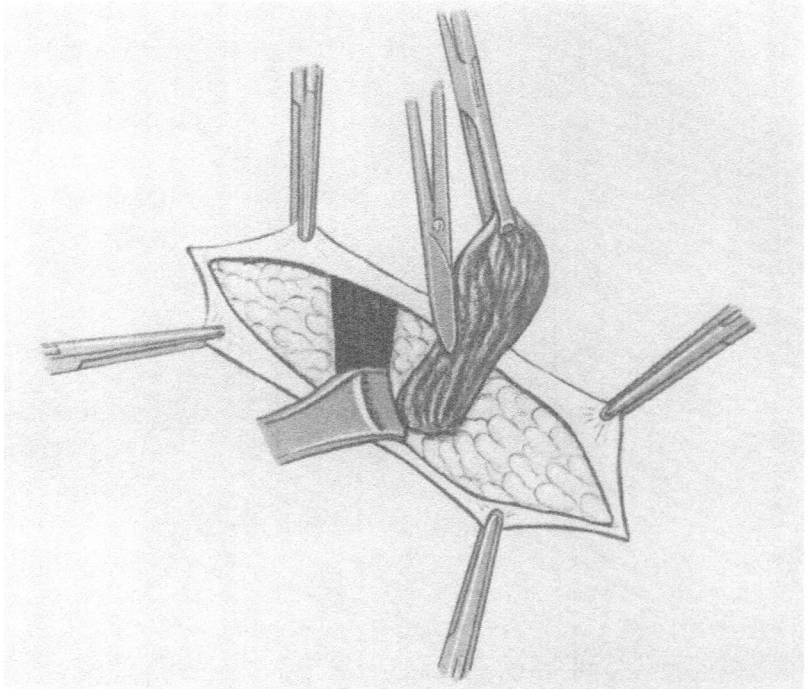

Figure 3. Dissection by hugging closely to peritoneal sac.

An Allis clamp then grasps the plug from the opposite side while the original Kelly clamp is removed. This creates an elegant tool for insertion of the mesh into the recurrent direct defect (Figure 4).

Interrupted 2-0 Novafil sutures fix the flat external end of the plug to the hernia margins using only about 3 mm of tissue for needle fixation. One suture should be inserted into the middle of the plug to prevent unraveling (Figures 5,6).

Recurrences of an indirect nature at the internal ring are demonstrated in these drawings. Once again, the plug is inserted in the same manner, using only 2 to 3 mm of defect margins to secure the plug on all sides except that of the spermatic cord. It does well when placed alongside the cord and has never done any damage to the cord (Figure 7). It should be noted here that the original descriptions of the plug in 1972 proved to be inaccurate since only two sutures were used and the plug was far too small.[3] Such a plug shrinks down to an inappropriate size and has therefore been replaced by a newer, much broader plug.

We are frequently asked why a patch is not used instead of a plug. A patch requires much wider dissection and therefore more tissue trauma. It creates a cul-de-sac behind the patch which can be the source of a new hernial defect. If a suture relaxes around the margins of a sewn patch, a recurrent hernia can result. The plug, by contrast, is solid, far more secure because of its shape and held firmly by 4 or 5 sutures.

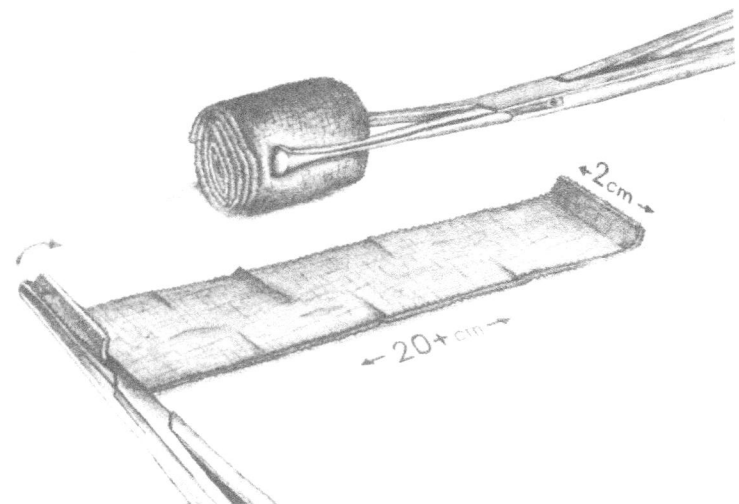

Figure 4. Creating the mesh plug.

POST-OPERATIVE COURSE

The patient may stand up and walk in about one hour and may have his breakfast or lunch. He is required to void normally and then goes home without restrictions. When he is seen 2-3 days later in the office, almost

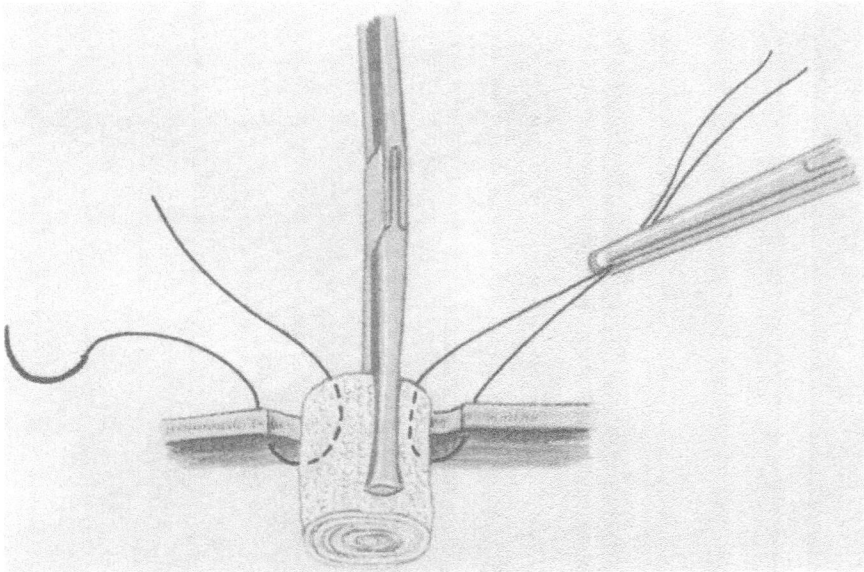

Figure 5. Insertion of plug.

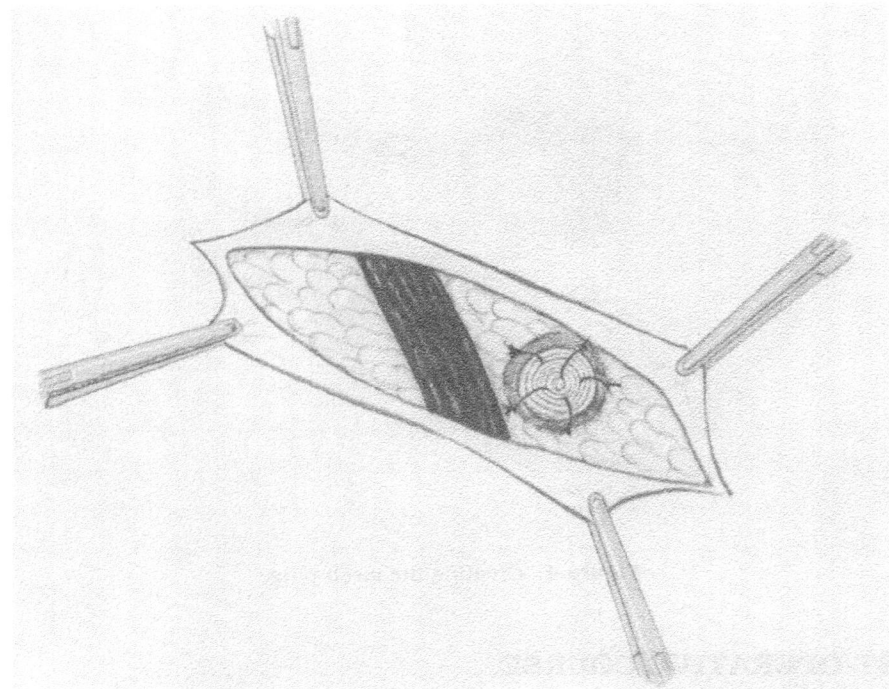

Figure 6. Completed suture of plug.

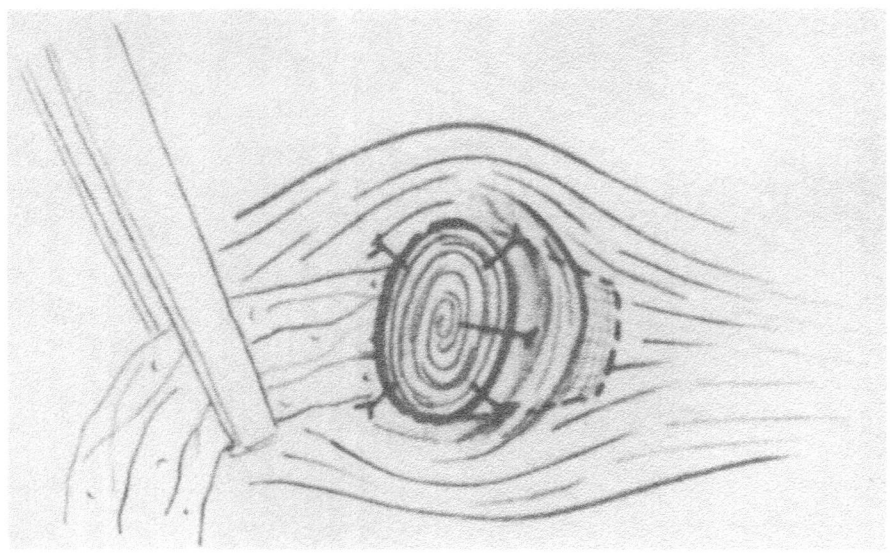

Figure 7. Plug next to cord for recurrent indirect hernia.

every patient makes the same comment declaring that "this was nothing compared to my last operation".

In 1989, we reported a 1.6 percent recurrence rate of 1,402 recurrent operations. At the present time, the number of our recurrences seems to be proportionately fewer.

APPROACH TO RECURRENT INGUINAL HERNIAS

Plans A, B, & C

While the plug repair is the preferred form of treatment, it is considered best for small recurrences (Plan A). For the small percentage of large defects such as that involving the entire canal floor, we employ Plan B.

To treat these larger defects, Plan B requires a wide sheet of mesh. In the presence of excessive scarring, anatomical landmarks may be seriously obscured. To reconstruct and discover recognizable landmarks, it is advisable to open the external oblique aponeurosis by beginning well lateral to the internal ring.

Here, in relatively virgin territory, the lower leaf of the external oblique is grasped and acts as a guide. Then, by hugging this lower lateral wall, it is relatively easy to identify Poupart's ligament and the pubic bone. To elevate the spermatic cord more safely, a curved hemostat under the cord, but hugging the pubic bone, is helpful. While dissecting up the cord, and if in doubt as to adjacent structures, it is advisable to include portions of the underlying tissues with the cord rather than to risk compromising the cord vessels. Any defect created by taking floor tissues will ultimately be covered by a wide sheet of mesh and made secure. Plan B requires freeing up of the entire cord up to the internal ring and then the application of mesh exactly as described for primary inguinal hernioplasty.

Plan C, is a properitoneal approach similar to that advocated by Stoppa and by Wantz.[4] By separating the muscle layers leading to the peritoneum, the latter is dissected free and a wide square sheet of mesh, about 15 cm in both directions, is inserted. It is fixed in place with 2 or 3 sutures and depends on intra-abdominal pressure to maintain it in place. This plan has had few indications for us except in extreme multiple recurrent hernias with hopelessly scarred anatomical findings. A recent article by Schaap et al[5] describes a 35 percent recurrence rate for recurrent hernias of patients treated via the open properitoneal approach suggesting the need for further improvement of that technique.

SUMMARY

The value of being able to cure recurrent hernias simply, even after numerous previous operations, is demonstrated. The plug approach provides a practical answer to meet the needs of the majority of patients with these frustrating problems.

REFERENCES

1. Greenburg AG: Revisiting the recurrent groin hernia. Am J Surg 1987;154:40.
2. Shulman Ag, Amid PK, Lichtenstein IL: The "plug" repair of 1,402 recurrent inguinal hernias. Arch Surg 1990;125:205-67.
3. Lichtenstein IL, Shore JM: Simplified repair of femoral and recurrent inguinal hernias by a "plug" technic. Am J Surg 1974; 128:439-44.
4. Wantz G: Personal experience with the Stoppa technique. In Nyhus LM, Condon RE. Hernia (3rd Edition). J.B. Lipincott, Philadelphia, PA, 1989:221-25.
5. Schaap HM, van de Pavoordt WM, Bast TJ: The properitoneal approach in the repair of recurrent inguinal hernias. Surg Gynecol Obstet 1992;174:460;-4.

OPEN TENSION-FREE REPAIR OF PRIMARY INGUINAL HERNIAS IN ADULT MALES

Alex G. Shulman, M.D.

Lichtenstein Hernia Institute
Los Angeles, California

The operative technique for tension-free hernia repair was initiated in 1984. All subsequent primary inguinal hernias in adult males were repaired in the manner to be described. Initially, the surgical community looked at this technique with justifiable suspicion. We now approach any discussion of this method with confidence based on results which have surpassed our most optimistic predictions.

The standard inguinal hernia repair results in an approximate 10 percent recurrence rate which includes 5 percent for indirect and 15 percent for direct hernias. With few exceptions, the recurrence rate remains the same throughout the world at the present time. The cause of recurrence is two-fold. In approximately 15 percent of males, there is a wide gap, 2 cm or larger, between the tendon of the transversus abdominis muscle and Poupart's ligament. Any attempt to bring the edges of these structures together may result in tension and early recurrence. Late recurrences are presumed to be caused by failure of collagen deposition in the fascia transversalis. Figures 1 and 2 display the anterior and posterior views of the inguinal anatomy described above.

The tension-free repair is an outpatient procedure performed under local anesthetic almost 100 percent of the time. The repair depends entirely upon a mesh prosthetic patch and there is no suture approximation of the edges of the hernial defect. The guiding principle is that recurrence may not occur through the mesh unless the mesh too small or too tight, i.e., around the edges of the mesh but never through it.

TECHNICAL SURGICAL POINTS

After infiltrating the skin and subcutaneous tissue with an anesthetic mixture (1:1 ratio) of 1% lidocaine and 0.5% bupivicaine), an approximate 5 to 6 cm long transverse skin incision is made extending laterally from the

Critical Issues in Surgery, Edited by A. C. Cernaianu et al.
Plenum Press, New York, 1995

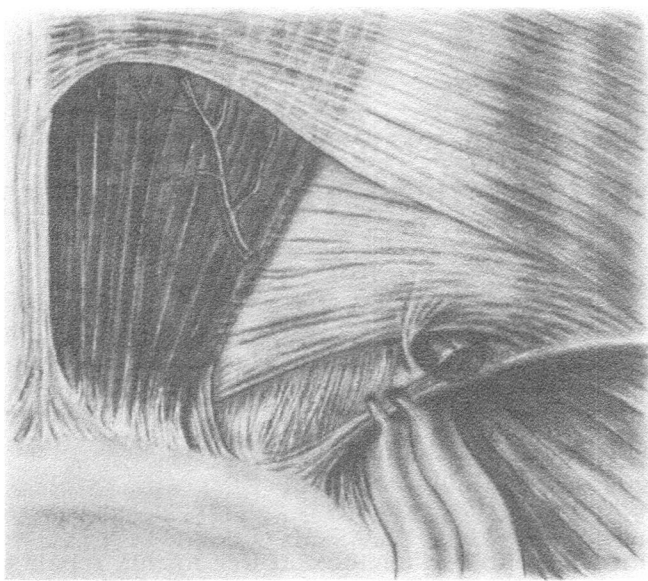

Figure 1. Posterior view of groin anatomy showing vulnerable area.

pubic tubercle. Approximately 8 cc of local anesthetic mixture is injected under the external oblique aponeurosis into the inguinal canal to block all three nerves. The ilioinguinal, genital branch of the genitofemoral, and the iliohypogastric nerves should be preserved. Under no circumstances should these entities be ligated as has been recommended as part of other procedures. This precaution prevents the occurrence of the chronic postoperative pain syndrome. The spermatic cord must be dissected completely from its floor, particularly over the pubic bone, to the level of the deep epigastric

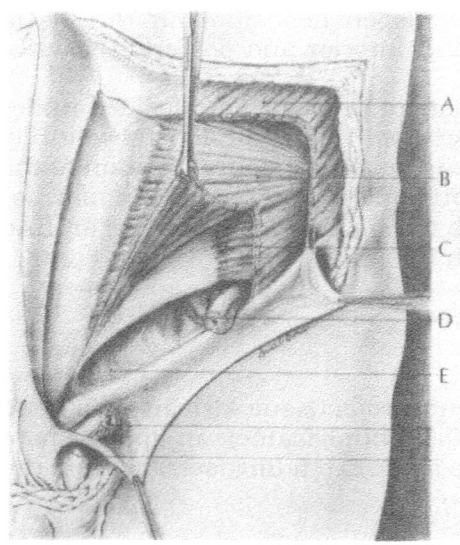

Figure 2. Anterior view of groin anatomy showing vulnerable area.

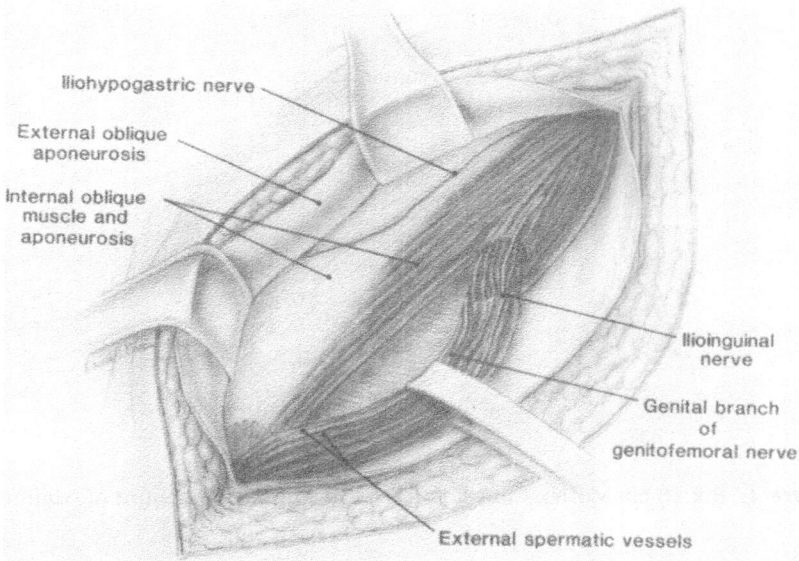

Figure 3. Freeing up of cord and minimal separation of cremaster fibers.

vessels. The cord should include the external spermatic vessels and the genital branch of the genitofemoral nerve, as well as the ilioinguinal nerve. It is unnecessary to widely dissect the cremaster fibers from the cord.

A small transverse incision, cutting the cremaster fibers, just at the level of the internal ring, will create a 1.5 to 2 cm gap when the internal oblique muscle retracts. This results in a narrowed cord only at the internal ring where it is needed. This avoids unnecessary excessive bleeding and trauma to the cord and testicular vasculonervous pedicle. Figure 3 demonstrates the retracted cord and the incised cremasteric fibers.

The indirect sac is identified and dissected from the spermatic cord and surrounding structures. Local anesthetic is generally injected into the base of the sac. The sac is then freed to the properitoneal level. Once it is opened, a finger is inserted to check for a possible femoral hernia. The open sac is then lowered into the peritoneal cavity without excision or ligation. In our combined experience, the sac has not been ligated in over 10,000 cases without adverse reaction. In the case of direct hernias, if the hernial bulge is slight, there should be nothing done to it. However, if the hernial sac is very large, it should be dissected down to its base and inverted with a light continuous absorbable suture.

MARLEX® MESH PROSTHESIS

Today Marlex® mesh (C.R. Bard, Inc., Bellerica, MA) is supplied in several different sizes. Most precut sheets of mesh are usually too small and cause the surgeon to adjust his operation to the sheet of mesh rather than tailoring the sheet of mesh to the operation. We therefore use the 8 cm X

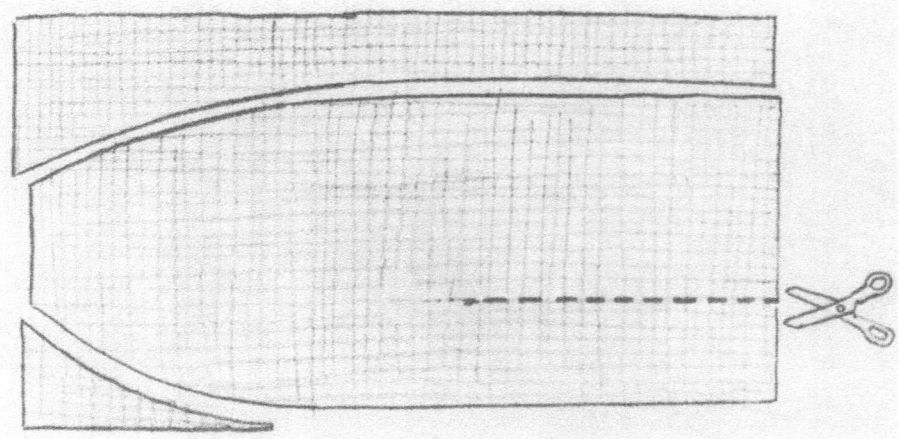

Figure 4. 8 x 16 cm Marlex® mesh patch - showing usual amount of trimming.

16 cm sheets which may require a minimal amount of tailoring to shape the defect (Figures 4,5).

The usual mesh is at least 6 cm wide. In the case of a very large patient, 7 to 8 cm wide may be employed. This type of mesh is preferred due to its tendency to become completely infiltrated by fibroblasts, its resistance to infection, hypoallergenicity and long record of success since first used in 1962.[1]

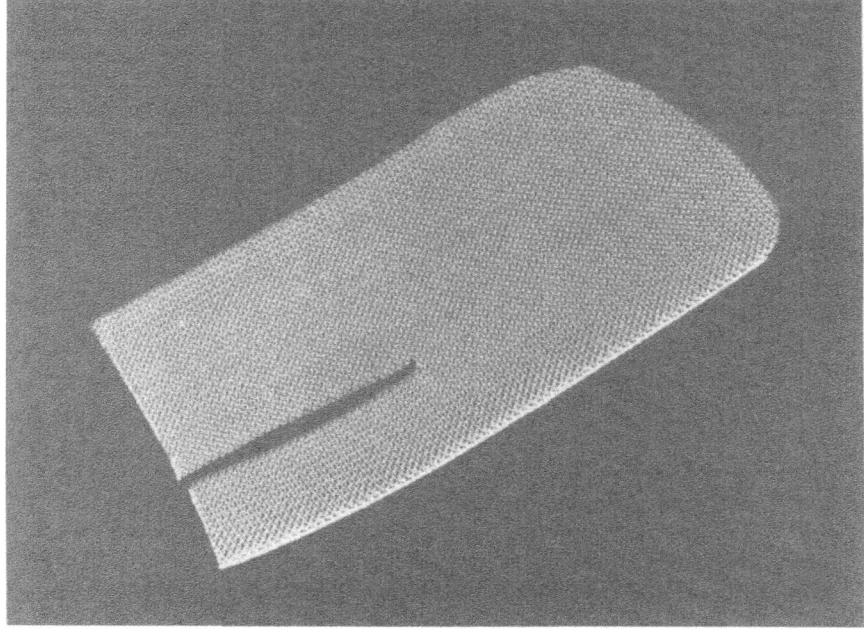

Figure 5. Photo of usual patch.

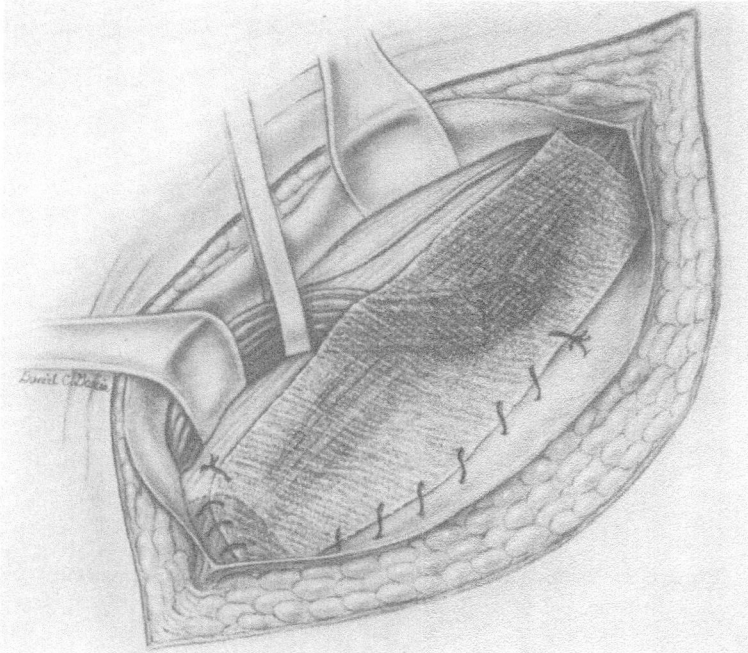

Figure 6. Patch sutured over pubic bone and to Poupart's ligament.

APPLICATION OF MESH

After clearing the pubic bone for a distance of 1.5 to 2 cm, the medial end of the mesh should be placed over this portion of the bone. In our experience, the only early failures were due to suturing the mesh to the side of the pubic bone rather than over it. This is probably the most critical point of the entire operation. Ingrowth of tissue over the pubis into the wide mesh application assures a strong area of fixation. In order to fix the medial and lower edges of the mesh in place, a continuous 2-0 Prolene or Novafil suture (monofilamented nonabsorbable) is started just medial and cephalad to the pubic bone to the soft tissues. The suture should lie on the bone but avoid the periosteum. The suture then continues into the shelving edge of Poupart's ligament and reaches as far as the internal ring where it is tied (Figure 6).

The lateral end of the mesh is now cut medially up to the internal ring, leaving two-thirds above and one-third below. Using a hemostat across but under the cord just distal to the internal ring, the upper leaf is placed under the cord in order for the mesh to straddle the cord when the mesh reaches its final position. The lateral tails of the mesh (the wide one over the narrow one) are held with a hemostat (Figure 7).

The upper leaf of the external oblique aponeurosis is retracted firmly to expose the underlying internal oblique muscle or aponeurosis as far medially as possible towards its junction with the rectus muscle. The mesh is laid flat on the internal oblique muscle and 4 or 5 interrupted 2-0

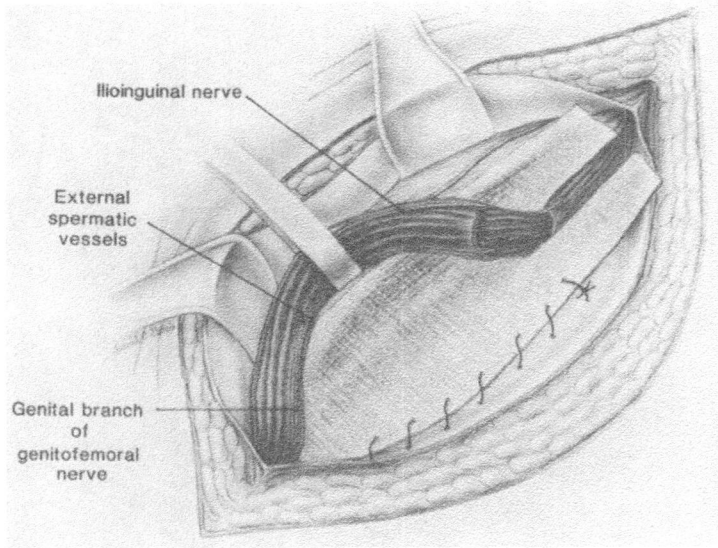

Figure 7. Medial end of mesh split and lying in final position.

absorbable sutures are placed to fix the mesh to the internal oblique muscle or aponeurosis. The most lateral suture should be at the level of the internal ring or just beyond it. This assures that the two tails will lie over each other, the wide one over the narrow one, lateral to the cord and not cross each other awkwardly (Figure 8).

At this point, one should determine how tight or how loose the mesh should be. The mesh lies absolutely flat, while the upper sutures are being placed and the external oblique aponeurosis is retracted. When the retractor is released the mesh buckles, spoiling the aesthetically pleasing smooth previous appearance of the mesh. However, it has been determined that this is desirable. The mesh should be loose and it should buckle, since this buckling will disappear as soon as the patient stands or coughs. Moreover, it is our observation that patients whose mesh is loose rather than tight have less postoperative discomfort.

CREATION OF THE NEW INTERNAL RING MADE OF MESH

A single suture of 2-0 Novafil or 2-0 Prolene grasps the shelving edge of Poupart's ligament lateral to the cord and then includes the lower margin of the lower tail and lower margin of the upper tail. When this is tied, a new internal ring made out of mesh is created (wide tail over narrow). The overlying of the tails create a sling comparable to the normal transversalis fascia sling (Figure 9).

The lateral ends of the tails are slightly shortened, if necessary, and then simply tucked laterally under the external oblique aponeurosis. The size of the new internal ring is evaluated. If too tight, two or three fibers of the mesh are simply incised to make it looser. If it is too loose, one suture

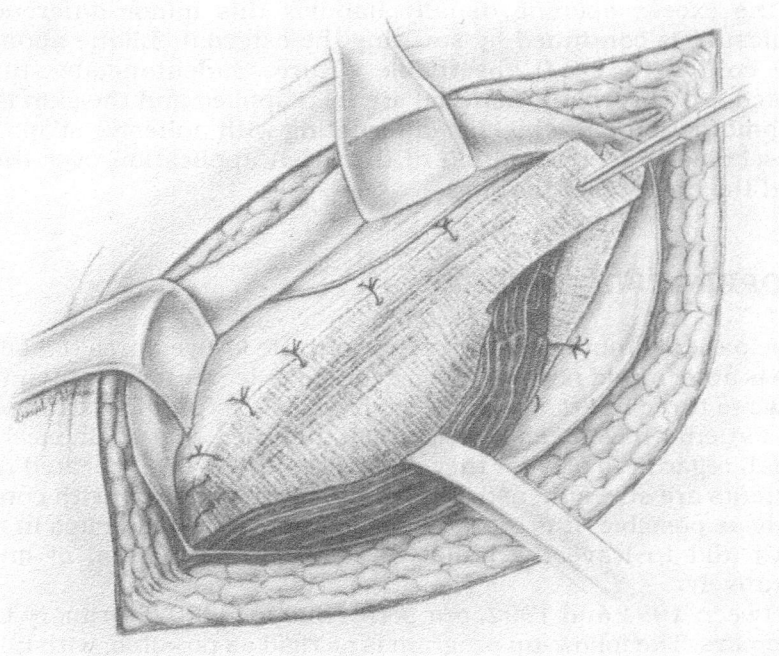

Figure 8. Medial upper sutures to internal oblique and mesh tails held in a clamp.

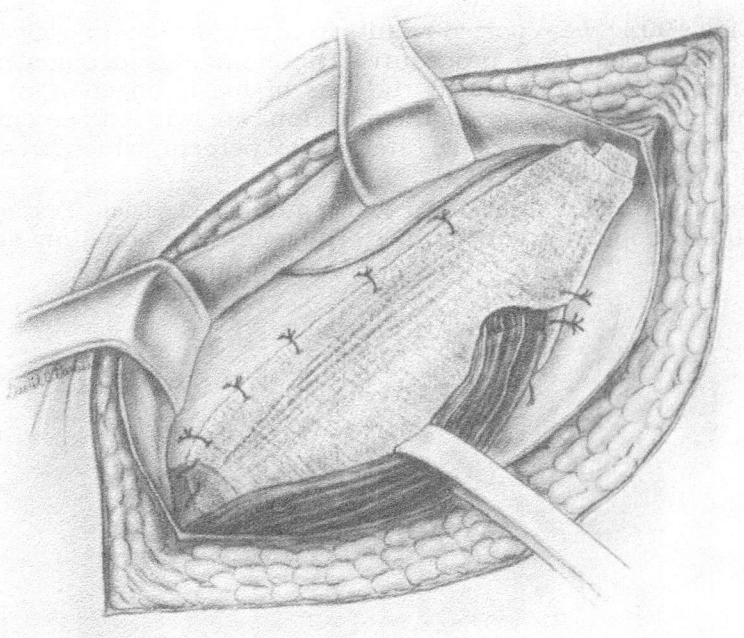

Figure 9. New internal ring of mesh created by a single suture of tail margins to Poupart's ligament.

closing the excess opening usually handles this minor difference. The wound closure is continued by suturing the external oblique aponeurosis over the cord with a 2-0 absorbable suture. Subcutaneous sutures of interrupted 3-0 absorbable material are then applied and the skin is closed with a combination of metal clips alternating with adhesive strips. Figure 10 is a schematic representation of the mesh application over the pubic bone and the creation of the ring.

POST-OPERATIVE COURSE

The patient ambulates within the hour. He is given breakfast or lunch and if he is able to void normally, is permitted to leave the outpatient facility within two to three hours. There are no physical restrictions to the patient's activity. Patients have been convincingly informed that their mesh repair will not fail regardless of what they do physically. By this repeated reassurance patients are strengthened to return to normal activity with confidence as quickly as possible. It is our practice to remove the skin clips in three or four days and to leave the adhesive strips on for a total of one week postoperatively.

Between 1984 and 1992, our series included 3,025 primary inguinal hernia repairs. The follow-up program is as rigid as possible, with no charge for post-operative visits for the rest of the patient's life. In case of a repair of any recurrence, there is no surgical fee for the patient. To date, there have only been 4 recurrences, mostly in the early years. Within the last five years, there have been no recurrences.

In May 1992,[2] we reported results from five different surgical groups using almost an identical procedure. These findings demonstrated the paucity of infections and ended the fear of mesh rejection in primary inguinal hernias. In these series, the infection rate was 0.3 percent with no rejections. The overall recurrence rate was 0.2 percent, which is essentially similar with our own.

Presently, we are witnessing a widely publicized series of experimental trials of laparoscopic herniorrhaphies. The technique is mainly advocated

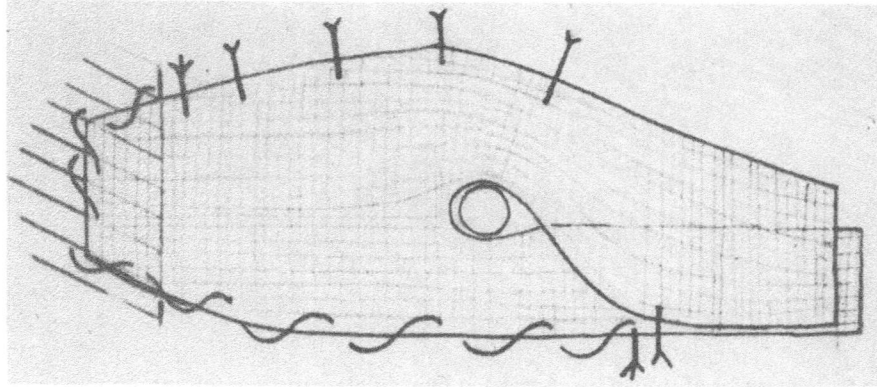

Figure 10. Schematic representation of suturing of mesh.

for lesser postoperative pain, and early ambulation and return to work for the highly motivated patients. When results from laparoscopic hernias are compared to the standard open operation, less pain is claimed for the laparoscopic procedure. However, there is no comparison between the laparoscopic technique and the tension-free repair. Those patients who volunteer for this experimental procedure of laparoscopic herniorrhaphy are usually highly motivated. They may return to work within 3 to 4 days. Our own highly motivated patients do likewise. In our series, we operated on numerous physicians and surgeons. Clinicians generally returned to make rounds on the first postoperative day and the surgeons returned to a full operating schedule within 3 to 4 days. By contrast, blue collar workers returned to work in 7 to 10 days. Prospective randomized studies may determine differences between laparoscopic hernia repair and the tension-free technique.

The lowest recurrence rates previously reported are from those undergoing the Shouldice repair. However, postoperative pain has been a recognized complication of the procedure.[3] In the course of repair with this technique, the genital branch of genitofemoral nerve is routinely ligated along with cremaster fibers. If the nerve is unusually large, it is expected that some of these patients may have chronic postoperative pain. As mentioned previously, the tension-free repair carefully protects all the nervous structures, there is no need to skeletonize the cord. In addition, the outcome of Shouldice repair depends on incorporating many layers of tissue for securing its strength. The tension-free repair uses one thin mesh sheet which achieves the same good results. Moreover, the operation performed under local anesthetic, in an outpatient setting with unlimited postoperative activity permitted, shorter disability time and less postoperative pain is an attractive technique. In addition, with a recurrence rate of approximately 0.4 percent in a patient population of over 23,000 operated by 77 surgeons, the goal of a 100 percent success in the repair of primary inguinal hernias in adults is now a realistic one.

REFERENCES

1. Amid PK, Shulman AG, Lichtenstein IL: Selecting synthetic mesh for the repair of groin hernia. Postgrad Gen Surg 1992;4:150-55.
2. Shulman AG, Amid PK, Lichtenstein IL: The safety of mesh repair for primary inguinal hernias. Am Surg 1992;58:255-57.
3. Tons HWCH, Kupczyk-Joeris D, Rotzscher VM, Schumpelick V: Chronic inguinal pain following Shouldice repair of primary inguinal hernias. Contemporary Surg 1990;37:24-30.

SEPSIS AND ITS RELATED DISORDERS: DEFINITIONS, EPIDEMIOLOGY, PATHOGENESIS AND PATHOPHYSIOLOGY

Bruce Friedman, M.D.

University of Medicine and Dentistry of New Jersey
Robert Wood Johnson Medical School at Camden
Cooper Hospital/University Medical Center
Camden, New Jersey

Sepsis and its related disorders, sepsis syndrome and shock, are the most common causes of death in the intensive care setting.[1] Recent advances in medicine have increased the risk of the sepsis syndromes. This has been attributed to several causes including frequent use of catheters and other invasive equipment, aggressive administration of oncologic chemotherapy, and the use of corticosteroids and other immunosuppressives in transplantation, inflammatory diseases and numerous other disorders.[2] This has placed a relatively large population of patients at high risk to develop sepsis and subsequent shock. In addition, improved medical care has lengthened the life span in the elderly and patients with immunodeficient, neoplastic and genetic/metabolic disorders, expanding their risk for infection and ultimately sepsis.

This chapter will examine the epidemiology, pathogenesis and physiology including a discussion of inflammatory mediators, cardiovascular dysfunction and disturbances in oxygen delivery, clinical organ manifestations, and finally management, treatment and future considerations regarding sepsis and its related disorders.

Before entering into a discussion of sepsis and septic shock, there must be an agreement in exactly what these terms represent. Until recently, the lack of precision in terms has hampered the progress of clinical study into the pathogenesis and physiology of sepsis and septic shock. In a landmark consensus conference, in 1991, the American College of Chest Physicians (ACCP) and the Society of Critical Care Medicine (SCCM) came together to develop definitions of the broad concept of sepsis to assist clinicians and researchers to better deal with sepsis and its sequelae.[3-4] A unifying new concept was developed which is labeled as the Systemic

Critical Issues in Surgery, Edited by A. C. Cernaianu et al.
Plenum Press, New York, 1995

51

Inflammatory Response Syndrome (SIRS) of which sepsis is only one causative factor. SIRS can be seen in association with a myriad of other noninfectious clinical conditions including pancreatitis, organ ischemia, multitrauma and tissue injury, hemorrhagic shock, immune-mediated organ injury and exogenous administration of putative mediators.[3] Sepsis becomes defined as the systemic inflammatory response to infection. This response is manifested by two or more conditions resulting from the infection which has been outlined in another chapter in this work. Septic Shock is then defined as sepsis with hypotension, despite adequate fluid resuscitation, along with the presence of perfusion abnormalities including, but not limited to, lactic acidosis, oliguria or acute alteration in mental status. Patients receiving vasopressors and/or inotropes may not be hypotensive, however, if perfusion abnormalities are present they are still considered within the boundaries of the definition. The ACCP/SCCM definitions provide a practical as well as a conceptual framework to improve early bedside detection and permit earlier intervention in sepsis as well as provide better communication between investigators researching the many aspects of this complicated disease state.

The most recently reported data indicates that sepsis is the thirteenth leading cause of death in the United States and accounts for five to ten billion dollars of health care costs annually.[5] The estimated mortality rate for sepsis, best defined generally as septicemia by the Center for Disease Control (CDC), is about 30 percent.[5] Establishing a true incidence of sepsis and its sequelae has been fraught with difficulty due to the lack of consensus on definitions and the inability to track related disorders since these are not recognized as reportable disease states (i.e., sepsis syndrome, SIRS, bacteremia, early vs. refractory septic shock). By the development of the ACCP/SCCM consensus definitions and their rapid acceptance by appropriate tracking organizations, i.e., CDC, Health Care Financing Agency (HCFA) these problems should resolve and improved statistical data will become available in the near future.

The current incidence of septic shock in the United States, estimated within the limitations noted above, is about 200,000 cases per year, of which 100,000 are fatal.[1] Statistically the incidence of sepsis and septic shock has increased to almost 150 percent of what it was ten years ago. Cases have risen from 75 to approximately 200 per 100,000 persons.[5] Independent of whether septic shock develops in the medical or surgical intensive care setting, a bad prognosis is inevitable in a large majority of cases. Mortality estimates range from 10 to 50 percent for patients that develop sepsis alone, to as high as 75 to 90 percent in those where sepsis becomes complicated with shock. Variations in definitions and the way in which the statistical data is collected may account for some of this variability. However, the high incidence and mortality as well as the health care costs demonstrates that there is still substantial need for research in these areas.

The most common etiology for sepsis and septic shock is infection. The source of infection usually presents clinically as pneumonia, vascular catheter infection, intraabdominal insult (i.e., cholecystitis, appendicitis, diverticulitis), soft tissue (i.e., decubitus ulcer or wound infection), or arising from the urinary tract. Other common causes include suppurative neurological disease (i.e., brain abscess, meningitis, subdural empyema), pyelonephritis, pelvic inflammatory disease, cellulitis or endocarditis. These diagnoses account for the majority of clinically apparent cases of sepsis.

Gram-negative bacteria are the most common and best studied organisms capable of triggering a septic host inflammatory response. The production of the potentially lethal microbial macromolecule, endotoxin, also referred to as lipopolysaccharide (LPS), by common gram negative organisms such as escherichia coli, pseudomonadaceae and enterobacteriaceae, stimulates the host immune system resulting in cellular activation and the release of various mediators of inflammation.[6] However, other microbial cell constituents from organisms such as gram-positive bacteria (staphylococcus aureus)[7], rickettsiae[8], fungi (candidemia)[9], viruses[10] and protozoa (malaria)[11], are also capable of inciting sepsis through the host response system. These highly pathogenic organisms produce compounds known as exotoxins which include Toxic Shock Syndrome Toxin-1 (TSST-1), hemolysins, leukocidin and streptolysins.[12] These lethal products are almost as potent as LPS in inciting an inflammatory response in the human host and are clinically and hemodynamically indistinguishable from endotoxin, at initial presentation.[13]

A similar sepsis-like response can arise in the absence of an infectious process.[14-15] Noninfectious causes of apparent sepsis have been recently classified under the term SIRS, which describes the inflammatory response, independent of its cause. Disorders such as burns, acute pancreatitis, anaphylaxis, acute intoxications or poisonings, vasculitides, heat stroke, graft rejection and extensive tissue injury/necrosis (i.e., rhabdomyolysis, mesenteric ischemia, crush injuries), will often be misdiagnosed as infectious mediated sepsis due to their almost identical clinical and hemodynamic presentation.[15] Thus, extensive tissue destruction activates a cascade of immunologic mediators suggesting that shock, multiple organ dysfunction/failure and death can arise from both, infectious and noninfectious causes.

The most common mechanism of sepsis is the proliferation of organisms within normally sterile body cavities after normal surface defenses have been breached.[16] The principle components involved are the tissue macrophages within the extensive reticuloendothelial system (90 percent in the liver as Kupffer cells) and noncellular mediators such as oxygen free radicals, nitric oxide and cytokines.[17-18] It appears that infectious mediated sepsis and non organism derived SIRS may share a common pathway in triggering the host immune response.

Gut, muscles, and skin represent most of the vascular beds in which vasoconstriction can occur in response to the catecholamine overload typical of early sepsis. Vascular shunting from the splanchnic beds, to provide vital visceral organ blood flow, may create gut dysfunction.[19] Due to the counter-current set-up of the vasculature near the tips of the intestinal villi and the right angle take-off of the villi vessels, nutrient artery blood flow is impaired and local tissue hypoxemia occurs.[20] The gut is uniquely predisposed and susceptible to the mucosal ischemia created by this decreased perfusional state. Compromise of the integrity of the gut mucosal barrier and translocation (leakage) of mediators and eventually intact organisms through the gut lining will occur.[21-23] Since all blood from the gut proceeds through the portal venous system, the liver is strategically placed behind the gut and must perform an important filtering function, removing endotoxin and other inflammatory mediators.[24-25] The sicker the patient, the more critical this filtering function becomes and the more likely that impaired hepatic clearance of septic by-products and Kupffer cell overload would occur.[22] Thus, a primary insult that results in gut dysfunction may be the common pathway for initiating, maintaining and prolonging the septic state to organ failure and death. The pathogenesis of sepsis must be viewed as a series of progressive events beginning with the failure of local integumentary, mucosal or pulmonary defenses to contain invading organisms and/or noninfectious inflammatory triggers. Rapidly following the release of septic by-products, such as endotoxin, into the bloodstream, a recently discovered complex cascade of highly interactive mediators has been found to cause profound damage to the vascular endothelium.[1,17] These microbial or complement activated stimuli stimulate mononuclear phagocytes (macrophage, mast cells) to release a wide array of soluble cytokines[26] including tumor necrosis factor alpha (TNF)[27-29], interleukin-1 (IL-1)[30-32], interleukin-6 (IL-6)[33], the phospholipid platelet activating factor (PAF)[34-35], and lipopolysaccharide binding protein (LBP). Concurrently, the complement and coagulation cascades can be triggered by LPS or other toxins. The cytokines, TNF, IL-1, and PAF, stimulate the arachidonic acid pathways in a variety of cells. This results in the production of endothelial damaging products including the leukotrienes, thromboxane A_2, and prostaglandins.[36]

Simultaneously, the neutrophils are recruited to the site of the inflammatory process by complement fragments (C5a) and their endothelial surface procoagulant activity and aggregation are enhanced by TNF and IL-1. In addition, the cytokines, including gamma interferon, increase neutrophil phagocytic activity and through the induction of the adhesion molecules intracellular adhesion molecule-1 (ICAM-1), endothelial adhesion molecule (ELAM-1) and vascular cell adhesion molecule (VCAM-1), prolong the neutrophil activation interval and promote endothelial-neutrophil adhesion.[37-38] Firm attachment to the endothelial lining is enhanced by LPS/cytokine activated neutrophil receptors, known as β_2 integrins (CD18, CD14, and CD11), interacting with the adhesion molecule ICAM-1.[39-40] Once the rapidly accumulated neutrophils attach to the endothelial lining, transendothelial migration at cell junctions and release of toxic neutrophilic products occurs. These activated leukocytes release oxygen free radicals (superoxide, myeloperoxidase, hydrogen peroxide and hydroxyl radicals) and lysosomal enzymes (proteases) which often cause severe damage to the vascular endothelium.[41-43] The combination of endothelial damage, creating large macromolecular cell gaps, and the transmigration of the neutrophils, allowing for accumulation in the subcellular regions, may lead to arteriolar damage. Along with PAF induced platelet aggregation, the leukocytes may form microemboli and maldistribution of blood flow occurs, resulting in organ tissue damage. This process is further enhanced by the potent vasoconstrictive effects of the leukotrienes, thromboxane and endothelin-1, and complement mediated cell lysis.[35,44]

Simultaneously, as the cascade of damaging events is underway, other mediators have been identified that may counterbalance these potentially lethal effects. In an attempt to restore hemostasis and repair and arrest the endothelial damage and curtail the mediator response, several endogenous proteins and cytokines are released. Endothelial derived relaxing factor (EDRF) and nitric oxide (NO) are generated via arginine metabolism by activated leukocytes and released from endothelial cells.[45] NO/EDRF are powerful vasodialators, altering microvascular tone, and also have strong antiaggregatory effects on platelets.[46] In combination with vasodilatory prostaglandins (PGI$_2$), histamine released from mast cell degranulation and PAF[35], NO/EDRF may counterbalance the maldistribution of blood flow and capillary block that occurs at the microvascular level.[46] Attenuation of cytokine effects have been shown with PGE$_2$, macrophage produced IL-8 and T cell derived IL-4 and IL-10.[47-50] These down regulating interleukins, along with platelet released transforming growth factor beta-1 (TGF-β_1), also inhibit endothelial-neutrophil adherence. Oxygen free radical toxicity can be inhibited by leukocyte-derived enzymatic antioxidants including superoxide dismutase and catalase and is suppressed by TGF-β_1.[51-52] Recently, a naturally occurring cationic antimicrobial protein, bacterial permeability increasing protein (BPI), has been identified in neutrophil azurophilic granules. It has several unique actions including surface binding to lipid A (the active moiety of endotoxin) downregulating the LPS response, suppression of cytokine production, and its sequence homology with lipopolysaccharide endotoxin binding protein (LBP) serves to curb the inflammatory response and reduce leukocyte adhesion. BPI may be a very important counterbalancing mediator in the sequential events surrounding the initial phases of sepsis.

These counterbalancing feedback mechanisms are often overwhelmed by the unyielding nature of the mediator driven inflammatory process. This is further complicated by both the autocrine nature of the mediator cascade, which allows each compound to stimulate release of each other, and the diversity of cell types that release these substances including the endothelial cells. Unchecked, the inflammatory process will disrupt and increase the permeability of the endothelium, cause direct cellular injury both locally and at additional organ sites, and ultimately, if uninterrupted, lead to multiple organ failure and death. The pathophysiologic consequences of this response include hemodynamic instability, alteration in vascular tone, cellular and organ injury that is perpetuated by tissue edema and hypoxia, and major alterations in oxygen consumption and delivery to cells and organs.

The physiologic response to invading microorganisms and the subsequent activation of the cascade of various mediators has profound effects on cardiovascular function.[2,53] Maldistribution of blood flow, endothelial destruction, and depression of myocardial contractility clinically translate into the most common hemodynamic responses in sepsis and shock, elevated cardiac output, reduced systemic vascular resistance (SVR) and compromised myocardial compliance (ejection fraction). Loss of vasoregulatory tone with vasodilation at the macrovascular level in the arterial circulation leads to the decline in the SVR.[54] At the capillary level there are alterations in blood flow patterns with arteriolar-venule beds being constricted, dilated and blocked by microthrombi. The decline in SVR leads to a fall in blood pressure, unless cardiac output can maintain systolic pressure. Hypotension ensues when venous return (preload) is compromised by excessive vasodilation, loss of circulating plasma volume or inadequate myocardial response/reserve makes elevation of cardiac output insufficient.[54] The myocardial response to sepsis and its related disorders is depressed ventricular contractility of both ventricles with compensatory dilation and consequently, reduced compliance ejection fraction.[55-56] Radionuclide cineangiography (MUGA) and pressure-volume performance plots in septic patients have demonstrated an increased end-diastolic volume, decreased EF and decreased stroke work index.[57-60] Stroke volume appears to be maintained and heart rate is elevated, thereby keeping cardiac output normal or increased in most patients. Ten percent of patients, despite adequate circulating blood volume may still present with myocardial dysfunction and low cardiac outputs. Prior ventricular dysfunction, overwhelming right ventricular overload and pulmonary hypertension, underlying poor medical condition and therefore altered physiologic responses, or excessive shock/mediator exposure manifested by rapid, irreversible organ failure may account for this abnormal response.[61] The pathophysiology that leads to impaired myocardial contractility had remained controversial until recently. Early animal data had suggested that myocardial performance may be impaired due to lowered coronary blood flow inducing ischemia and myocardial dysfunction. However, coronary flow was directly measured in human subjects with sepsis revealing normal to improved flow, compared to controls, and no differences in lactate extraction from the coronary blood.[62] Ischemic myocardial dysfunction was effectively excluded as an explanation. Alternatively, a myocardial depressive substance had been postulated and subsequently experimentally and clinically demonstrated.[63-64] In vitro myocytes, exposed to the serum of septic patients, undergo marked depression.[63] The true identity of this elusive substance has not been completely verified. It is clearly induced by endotoxin exposure in normal volunteers, elevated by IL-1, and clinically mimicked by TNF.[65] The reversible nature of the cardiac dysfunction that occurs in septic shock suggests that the presence of a myocardial depressive cytokine, or other mediator, may explain the pathophysiologic response to sepsis. Prolongation of the impaired cardiac performance may also be contributed by the presence of cardiac edema, leading to cellular damage, post aggressive plasma volume resuscitation. More investigation into this phenomenon is underway.

Despite the therapeutic interventions to maintain normal blood pressure gradients and acceptable cardiac outputs, there is a large body of evidence suggesting that the systemic distribution of blood flow is maldistributed and that energy substrate and oxygen utilization may be impaired.[66-67] Under normal conditions whole body oxygen consumption (VO_2) and oxygen delivery (DO_2), the product of cardiac output and arterial oxygen content (CaO_2, Hb), are independent variables. However, in sepsis and shock, the body's metabolic demands increase markedly. VO_2 elevates, but extraction of oxygen by tissues from arterial blood is impaired as a result of tissue hypoxia and maldistribution of micro/macrocirculations.[68] The combination of increased metabolic demands and distributive abnormalities leads to increases in anaerobic threshold with VO_2 dependent on DO_2. Due to the vasoconstriction, endothelial damage and damaged microvasculature, resulting from extensive mediator release, oxygenated arterial blood may supply tissues that do not require blood flow to sustain metabolism yet provide inadequate nutrient flow to areas heavily dependent on aerobic metabolism. Clinically this manifests as high cardiac outputs, above normal DO_2, and a high mixed venous oxygen saturation (SvO_2) indicative of a low tissue extraction of oxygen.[69] In the presence of inadequate tissue perfusion, impaired extraction and marked microvascular shunting to many cellular and systemic organ beds, a systemic lactic acidosis is not uncommonly found. Lactic acid, along with DO_2 potentially appear to be markers of survival in the patient with septic shock.[69-70] Nonsurvivors are consistently seen when lactates are greater than 10 mmol/L and DO_2 is unable to be maintained at greater than 15 mL/min/kg.[69-71] Certain cytokines, specifically interleukin-6 (IL-6) have also shown remarkable consistency with respect to survival vs. nonsurvival as well as being a marker of the progression and eventual improvement of the septic process.[33,72] This specific attribute of IL-6 may allow us to use it as a research tool, applying it as an endpoint, by serially following its patterns, throughout the septic course, during various clinical anticytokine or other mediator trials.

The failure of oxygen extraction, characteristic of sepsis and shock, may also be due to direct histotoxic injury, rendering cells incapable of oxygen utilization. Several animal models of septic shock have demonstrated that endotoxin and other early mediators (TNF, IL-1) may cause uncoupling of oxidative phosphorylation.[73] If aerobic metabolism is impaired by either direct inhibition of the mitochondrial cellular metabolism, through impaired DO_2/VO_2 due to microcirculatory alterations or by cellular edema from capillary and endothelial leak as a result of mediator triggered responses and aggressive fluid resuscitation, anaerobic metabolism will predominate. The inefficiency of anaerobism decreases the energy production of the cell from 36 ATP to 2 ATP molecules. This leads to an increased production of pyruvate and consequently lactate and an acidic cellular environment.[74] In the setting of hypermetabolic septic shock the energy demands to maintain cellular membrane integrity will eventually, and sometimes rapidly, go unmet. Consequently, cell lysis, death and ultimately a progression to partial then complete organ failure occurs.

Recently, these concepts of tissue hypoxia and bioenergetics (loss of aerobic metabolism) have been challenged by some elegant scientific data presented by Hotchkiss and Karl.[75] They suggest that the generation of lactate does not necessarily reflect cellular hypoxia. Lactic acid elevations may be the result of protein degradation and elevated glycolysis with increased production of pyruvate but an unchanged pyruvate/lactate ratio. Biochemically, this does not translate into a change to anaerobic metabolism. Also, there has been no human data demonstrating an alteration in phosphorylation by endotoxin or other mediators, predisposing toward anaerobic metabolism. Through a sophisticated phosphate labeled nuclear magnetic resonance scan, in a septic animal model, they were unable to show any loss of ATP at the individual cellular level.[75] Furthermore, using the same model, a measurement of cellular hypoxia, utilizing a highly oxygen specific (F)fluoromisonidazole compound, revealed no evidence of tissue hypoxia in gastrocnemius, heart, lung, brain or diaphragm.[75] They postulate, based on these findings, that DO_2/VO_2 dependency may represent the normal physiologic response of the system rather than an abnormal manifestation of impaired O_2 extraction. Although this is quite provocative data, it is heavily dependent on technically difficult animal data. Also skeletal muscle, and potentially other human organs, can sustain dramatic alterations in DO_2 without evidence of cellular hypoxia. Available human clinical data has demonstrated outcome may be improved with manipulation of oxygen delivery and that survivability may be heavily dependent on the reversal of high lactic acid states.[69,71] Thus, this exciting new challenge to our current pathophysiologic concepts does not offer alternate explanations to present clinical data.

In summary, an understanding of the complex mechanisms involved with the initiation and progression of sepsis and shock and the application of new and more concise definitions of terms will improve overall patient care in the intensive care unit. Furthermore, as more sophisticated technological and pharmaceutical manipulations of the septic process are developed and brought to clinical trial, the clinician will need a thorough comprehension of the pathogenesis and pathophysiology of sepsis. The research potential is exciting and abundant, and the future impact on patient morbidity and mortality remains substantial.

REFERENCES

1. Bone RC: The pathogenesis of sepsis. Ann Int Med 1991;115:457-469.
2. Parillo JE, Parker MM, Natanson C, Sufferidni AF, Danner RL, Cunnion RE, Ognibene FP: Septic shock in humans: advances in the understanding of the pathogenesis, cardiovascular dysfunction, and therapy. Ann Int Med 1990;113:227-242.
3. ACCP/SCCM Consensus Conference. Definitions for sepsis and organ failure and guidelines for the use of innovative therapies in sepsis. Chest 1992;101:1644-1655.
4. SCCM/ACCP Consensus Conference. Definitions for sepsis and organ failure and guidelines for the use of innovative therapies in sepsis. Crit Care Med 1992;20:864-874.
5. Angus DC, Kramer DJ: Bacteremia and sepsis: clinical perspectives. In: Pinsky MR, Dhainout JEA eds. Pathophysiologic foundations of critical care. Williams & Wilkins, Baltimore, MD, 1993:96-111.
6. Light RB: Approach to sepsis of unknown origin. In: Hall JB, Schmidt GA, Wood LDH eds. Principles of critical care. New York: McGraw-Hill, 1992:1159-1171.
7. Sheagren JN: Staphylococcus aureus: the persistent pathogen. NEJM 1984;310:1368-1372.
8. Hattwick MAW, Retailliau H, O'Brien RJ: Fatal rocky mountain spotted fever. Arch Int Med 1978;240:1499-1503.
9. Rutledge R, Mandel SR, Wild RE: Candida species: insignificant contaminant or pathogenic species. Ann Surg 1986;52:299-304.
10. Okrent DJ, Winston AE: Cardiorespiratory patterns in viral septicemia. Am J Med 1987;83:681-686.
11. Smit WM, van Straaten HMO, Zandstra DF: Fulminant falciparum malaria. Int Care Med 1990;16:517-519.
12. Danner RL, Sufferdini AF, Natanson C, Parillo JE: Microbial toxins: role in the pathogenesis of septic shock and multiple organ failure. In: Bihari DJ, Cerra FB eds. Multiple organ failure. Fullerton, CA: SCCM, 1989:151-191.
13. Ahmed AJ, Kruse JA, Haupt MJ, Chandrasekar PH, Carlson RW: Hemodynamic responses to gram-positive versus gram-negative sepsis in critically ill patients with and without circulatory shock. Crit Care Med 1991;19:1520-1525.
14. DeCamp MM, Demling RH: Posttraumatic multisystem organ failure. JAMA 1988;260(4):530-533.
15. Cerra FB: Multiple organ failure syndrome. Dis-a-Month 1992;38(12):843-895.
16. Light RB: Sepsis syndrome. In: Hall JB, Schmidt GA, Wood LDH eds. Principles of critical care. McGraw-Hill, New York, NY, 1992:645-661.
17. Bone RC. Sepsis syndrome, part 1: the diagnostic challenge. J Crit Ill 1991;6(6):525-539.
18. Filkins JP: Cytokines, mediators of the septic syndrome and septic shock. In: Taylor RW, Shoemaker WC, eds. Critical care state of the art. SCCM, Fullerton, CA, 1991;(12):351-370.

19. Carrico CJ, Meakins JL, Marshall JC: Multi-organ-failure syndrome. Arch Surg 1986;121:196-200.
20. Shepard AP, Kiel JW: A model of countercurrent shunting of oxygen in the intestinal villus. Am J Physiol 1992;262:H1136-1142.
21. Deitch EA, Winerton J, Bey R. The gut as the portal of entry for bacteremia. Ann Surg 1987;205:681-692.
22. Wells CL, Maddus MA, Simmons RL: Proposed mechanisms for the translocation of intestinal bacteria. Rev Infect Dis 1988;10(5):958-979.
23. Mainous MR, Deitch EA. Bacterial translocation and its potential role in the pathogenesis of multiple organ failure. J Intensive Care Med 1992;7:101-108.
24. Matuschak GM, Rinaldo JE, Pinsky MR: Effect of end-stage liver failure on the incidence and resolution of the adult respiratory distress syndrome. J Crit Care 1987;2:162-173.
25. Pinsky MR, Matuschak GM: Multiple systems organ failure Crit Care Clin 1989;5(2):199-220.
26. Tracey KJ, Lowry SF: The role of cytokine mediators in septic shock. Adv Surg 1990;23:21-56.
27. Simpson SQ, Casey LC: Role of tumor necrosis factor in sepsis and acute lung injury. Crit Care Clin 1989;5(1):27-47.
28. Franzoni G, Leech J, Jensen G, Brotman S: Tumor necrosis factor alpha: what role in sepsis and organ failure? J Crit Ill 1991;6:796-805.
29. Hinshaw LB, Tekamp-Olson P, Chang ACK, Lee PA, Taylor FB, Murray CK, et.al: Survival of primates in LD_{100} septic shock following therapy with antibody to tumor necrosis factor. Circ Shock 1990;30:279-292.
30. Damas P, Reutter A, Gysen P, Demonty J Lamy M, Franchimont P: Tumor necrosis factor and interleukin-1 serum levels during severe sepsis in humans. Crit Care Med 1989;17:975-978.
31. Cannon JG, Tompkins RG, Gelfand JA, Michie HR, Stanford GG, van der Meer JWM, et.al: Circulating interleukin-1 and tumor necrosis factor in septic shock and experimental endotoxin fever. JID 1990;161:79-84.
32. Dinarello CA, Wolff SM: The role of interleukin-1 in disease. N Engl J Med 1993;328:106-113.
33. Hack CE, De Groot ER, Felt-Bersma JF, Nuijens JH, Van Schijndel RJMS, Eerenberg-Belmer AJM, et.al: Increased plasma levels of interleukin-6 in sepsis. Blood 1989;74(5):1704-1710.
34. Chang SW: Endotoxin-induced lung vascular injury: role of platelet activating factor, tumor necrosis factor and neutrophils. Clin Research 1991;39:528-536.
35. Koltai M, Hosford D, Braquet PG: Platelet-activating factor in septic shock. New Horizons 1993;1(1):87-95.
36. Ball HA, Cook JA, Wise C, Halushka PV: Role of prostaglandins and leukotrienes in endotoxic and septic shock. Int Care Med 1986;12:116-126.
37. Lo SK, Everitt J, Gu J, Malik AB: Tumor necrosis factor mediates experimental pulmonary edema by ICAM-1 and CD18-dependent mechanisms. J Clin Invest 1992;89:981-988.
38. Vedder NB, Fouty BW, Winn RK, Harlan JM, Rice CL: Role of neutrophils in generalized reperfusion injury associated with resuscitation from shock. Surgery 1989;106:509-516.
39. Vedder NB, Winn RK, Rice CL, Chi EY, Arfors KE, Harlan JM: A monoclonal antibody to the adherence-promoting leukocyte glycoprotein, CD18, reduces organ injury and improves survival from hemorrhagic shock and resuscitation in rabbits. J Clin Invest 1988;81:939-944.
40. Arnaout MA: Structure and function of the leukocyte adhesion molecules CD11/CD18. Blood 1990;75(5):1037-1050.
41. Nahum A, Sznajder JI: Role of free radicals in critical illness. In: Hall JB, Schmidt GA, Wood LDH eds. Principles of Critical Care. McGraw-Hill, New York, NY, 1992:679-692.
42. Robinson MK, Rounds JD, Hong RW, Jacobs DO, Wilmore DW: Glutathione deficiency increases organ dysfunction after hemorrhagic shock. Surgery 1992;112:140-149.
43. Warren JS, Ward PA: Review: oxidative injury to the vascular endothelium. Am J Med Sci 1986;292(2):97-103.

44. Henrich WL: The endothelium—a key regulator of vascular tone. Am J Med Sci 1991;302:319-328.

45. Snyder SH, Bredt DS: Biological roles of nitric oxide. Sci Am May, 1992:68-77.

46. Vallance P, Moncada S: Role of endogenous nitric oxide in septic shock. New Horizons 1993;1(1):77-86.

47. Malefyt RW, Abrams J, Bennett B, Figdor CG, de Vries JE: Interleukin 10 (IL-10) inhibits cytokine synthesis by human monocytes: an autoregulatory role of IL-10 produced by monocytes. J Exp Med 1991;174:1209-1220.

48. Ralph P, Nakoinz I, Sampson-Johannes A, Fong S, Lowe D, Min HY, Lin L: IL-10, T lymphocyte inhibitor of human blood cell production of IL-1 and tumor necrosis factor. J Immunology 1992;148(3):808-814.

49. Bogdan C, Vodovotz Y, Nathan C: Macrophage deactivation by interleukin 10. J Exp Med 1991;174:1549-1555.

50. Fiorentino DF, Zlotnik A, Mosmann TR, Howard M, O'Garra A. IL-10 inhibits cytokine production by activated macrophages. J Immunology 1991;147(11):3815-3822.

51. Shindoh C, Dimarco A, Nethery D, Supinski: Effect of PEG-superoxide dismutase on the diaphragmatic response to endotoxin. Am Rev Respir Dis 1992;145:1350-1354.

52. Koyama S, Kobayashi T, Kubo K, Sekiguchi M, Ueda G. Recombinant superoxide dismutase attenuates endotoxin-induced lung injury in awake sheep. Am Rev Respir Dis 1992;145:1404-1409.

53. Snell RJ, Parillo JE: Cardiovascular dysfunction in septic shock. Chest 1991;99:1000-1009.

54. Groeneveld ABJ, Bronsveld W, Thijs LG: Hemodynamic determinants of mortality in human septic shock. Surgery 1986;99(2):140-152.

55. Parker MM, McCarthy KE, Ognibene FP, Parillo JE: Right ventricular dysfunction and dilatation similar to left ventricular changes, characterize the cardiac depression of septic shock in humans. Chest 1990;97:126-131.

56. Parker MM, Shelhamer JH, Bacharach SL: Profound but reversible myocardial depression in patients with septic shock. Ann Int Med 1984;100:483-490.

57. Parker MM, Shelhamer JH, Natanson C, Alling DW, Parillo JE: Serial cardiovascular variables in survivors and nonsurvivors of human septic shock: heart rate as an early predictor of prognosis. Crit Care Med 1987;15:923-929.

58. Parker MM, Sufferdini AF, Natanson C, Ognibene FP, Shelhamer JH, Parillo JE: Responses of left ventricular function in survivors and nonsurvivors of septic shock. J Crit Care 1989;4:19-25.

59. Parillo JE: The cardiovascular response to human septic shock. In: Furhman BP, Shoemaker WC eds. Critical care: state of the art. SCCM, Fullerton, CA, 1989;(10):285-314.

60. Sufferdini AF, Fromm PE, Parker MM: The cardiovascular response of normal humans to the administration of endotoxin. N Engl J Med 1989;321:280-287.

61. Jardin F, Brun-Ney D, Auvert B, Beauchet A, Bourdarias JP: Sepsis-related cardiogenic shock. Crit Care Med 1990;18:1055-1060.

62. Cunnion RE, Schaer GL, Parker MM, Natanson C, Parillo JE: The coronary circulation in human septic shock. Circulation 1986;73:637-644.

63. Parillo JE, Burch C, Shelhamer JH, Parker MM, NatansonC, Schuette W: A circulating myocardial depressant substance in humans with septic shock: septic shock patients with a reduced ejection fraction have a circulating factor that depresses in vitro myocardial performance. J Clin Invest 1985;76:1539-1553.

64. Reilly JM, Cunnion RE, Burch-Whitman C, Parker MM, Shelhamer JH, Parillo JE. A circulating myocardial depressant substance is associated with cardiac dysfunction and peripheral hypoperfusion (lactic acidemia) in patients with septic shock. Chest 1989;95:1072-1080.

65. Hollenberg SM, Cunnion RE, Lawrence M, Kellet JL, Parillo JE: Tumor necrosis factor depresses myocardial cell function: results using an in vitro assay of myocyte performance. Clin Res 1989;37:528A.

66. Harkema JM, Dean RE, Stephan RN, Chaudry IH: Cellular dysfunction in sepsis. J Crit Care 1990;5(1):62-69.

67. Shoemaker WC, Appel PL, Kram HB: Role of oxygen debt in the development of organ failure sepsis, and death in high risk surgical patients. Chest 1992;102:208-215.

68. Rackow EC, Astiz ME, Weil MH: Cellular oxygen metabolism during sepsis and shock. JAMA 1988;259(13):1989-1993.

69. Tuchscmidt J, Fried J, Swinney R, Sharma OP: Early hemodynamic correlates of survival in patients with septic shock. Crit Care Med 1989;17:719-723.

70. Bakker J, Coffernils M, Leon M, Gris P, Vincent JL: Blood lactate levels are superior to oxygen-derived variables in predicting outcome in human septic shock. Chest 1991;99:956-962.

71. Tuchschmidt J, Fried J, Astiz M, Rackow E: Elevation of cardiac output and oxygen delivery improves outcome in septic shock. Chest 1992;102:216-220.

72. Schluter B, Konig B, Bergmann U, Muller FE, Konig W: Interleukin 6: a potential mediator of lethal sepsis after major thermal trauma: evidence for increased IL-6 production by peripheral blood mononuclear cells. J Trauma 1991;31(12):1663-1670.

73. Astiz M, Rackow EC, Weil MH, Schumer W: Early impairment of oxidative metabolism and energy production in severe sepsis. Circ Shock 1988;26:311-320.

74. Mizock B: Septic shock: a metabolic perspective. Arch Int Med 1984;144:579-585.

75. Hotchkiss RS, Karl IE: Reevaluation of the role of cellular hypoxia and bioenergetic failure in sepsis. JAMA 1992;267:1503-1510.

THE SEPTIC PATIENT: FUTURE DIRECTIONS

T. James Gallagher, M.D.

University of Florida College of Medicine
Shands Hospital
Gainesville, Florida

In order to provide some insights into potential new therapies for sepsis, we must contend with a new terminology proposed by a joint consensus conference of the Society of Critical Care Medicine and the American College of Chest Physicians. *Systemic Inflammatory Response Syndrome* (SIRS) describes the body's widespread response to inflammation. Sepsis is a subcategory for those with documented infection. *Multiple Organ Dysfunction Syndrome* is the reflection of the degree of organ damage from the systemic inflammatory response syndrome.[1] This can be direct or indirect injury.

In the last decade, the reported death rate for patients with ARDS has decreased from approximately 80 to 50 percent.[2] The terminology *ARDS* does not define a specific disease process. Instead, the lung demonstrates a generalized response and clinical appearance, to various etiologies. Changes ascribed to ARDS can and do in fact represent other clinical conditions. Examples might include lung infection and/or pneumonia, decreased fractional residual capacity (FRC) as may occur following upper abdominal or intrathoracic surgery, aspiration syndrome, or inhalation of various noxious substances. This author contends that a diagnosis of ARDS should be reserved for those conditions in which the aforementioned

Table 1. Systemic Inflammatory Response Syndrome

Temperature	< 36–C > 38–C
Heart rate	> 90/min.
Respiration	> 20/min.
$PaCO_2$	< 32 mmHg
WBC	< 4,000 > 12,000
BANDS	> 10%

Critical Issues in Surgery, Edited by A. C. Cernaianu et al.
Plenum Press, New York, 1995

pulmonary response follows generalized sepsis, sepsis syndrome, or multiple organ failure.

True sepsis-associated ARDS represents an increase in extravascular lung water, decreased oxygenation as indicated by various parameters including PaO_2, $PaCO_2/FiO_2$ ratio and venous admixture.[3] All the while, pulmonary capillary wedge pressure remains within normal range; this is defined as noncardiogenic pulmonary edema. During this state, fluid enters the lung through the endothelial cell junctions. The lung primarily remains in a dry state by means of lymphatic drainage which removes the fluid as it enters the interstitial space. During sepsis it seems that contraction develops in the endothelial cells, thereby widening these intercellular clefts. Since flow is related to the fourth power of the radius, a significant change in the diameter of these gaps can result in large influxes of fluid into the interstitial space; far in excess of what can be removed by lymphatic drainage alone. Fluid then first fills the interstitial space and finally the alveolar compartments. Studies by Brigham, et al[4], have indicated that as microvascular pressures increase under conditions of altered permeability, fluid accumulation far exceeds that which develops when pressure increases alone, without evidence of increased altered permeability.

In recent years it has become clear that antimicrobial agents directed against the gram negative organisms have been less than completely successful. Efforts have now focused on the bacteria products such as, cell wall endotoxin.[5] Data would suggest that in those septic patients in whom endotoxemia was present, irrespective of the blood level, the incidence of ARDS appeared to be significantly higher than in those in whom endotoxin was not isolated.[6] Likewise, the presence of endotoxin was associated with a greater incidence of renal failure, and greater use of vasopressors. Further subdivision of patients into those with positive blood cultures demonstrated that those with endotoxin present had a significantly higher mortality rate. Also, the incidence of ARDS and renal failure was increased.

Monoclonal antibody to the lipid moiety of endotoxin heralded the first breakthrough.[7] However, at this writing, the early promise held out for these agents has been dimmed by what to some seems to be inconclusive and non-convincing results. This in turn has spurred on efforts directed at specific cytokines.

The release of endotoxin ultimately stimulates the release of other cytokines, such as tumor necrosis factor (TNF), IL-6 and IL-1. TNF is generally associated with the immune system, and acts as an intercellular communicator. Clinical changes including hypotension, altered perfusion, and reduced cardiac output develop in association with elevated TNF levels.[8] Studies have demonstrated that when TNF is present in septic patient, irrespective of the blood level, the death rate is considerably higher than in those patients in which TNF has not been detected.[9] It appears to make little difference if infection is noted in blood, sputum or other areas. TNF has been implicated in the direct alteration of capillary permeability.[10] Animal studies with monoclonal antibodies to TNF can prevent the usual hemodynamic and pulmonary responses caused by this cytokine.[11] It remains unclear what the normal relationship of the TNF response is to sepsis. Does the appearance of TNF simply reflect overwhelming sepsis and continued stimulation of TNF release, or in fact does the actual TNF level itself have some impact on the ultimate outcome of these patients?

Another cytokine, IL-1, also appears to be an important mediator of the septic response.[12] It exists as IL-1α and IL-1β.[13,14] Both cytokines bind to the same receptor. The activity of each may be somewhat different. IL-1 has many of the same biologic activates as TNF. These include capillary leak, endothelial cell activation, pulmonary congestion and T & B cell activation. Symptoms related to IL-1 include fever, myalgia, hypotension and myocardial depression. TNF and IL-1 together apparently act to release IL-6, which increases in response to endotoxin, which in turn stimulates IL-1 release. Both cytokines can respond in multiple bursts to endotoxin presence. IL-6 may serve more as a marker of earlier presence of TNF and IL-1. Many of these clinical manifestations can be prevented by cyclooxygenase inhibitors. This would indicate a role for prostaglandin mediation of circulating IL-1. Clinical studies have begun to test the role of IL-1 receptor antagonists in aiding the prevention of many of the usual responses to sepsis and endotoxin.

Another mediator, platelet activating factor (PAF) is derived from neutrophils, eusinophils monocytes, macrophages, platelets, and endothelial cells. PAF has been associated with bronchial constriction, as well as dilatation and constriction of both, the pulmonary and systemic beds. PAF may ultimately lead to altered vascular permeability.[15] In addition to reduced capillary integrity in the lung and elsewhere, PAF may stimulate platelet aggregation, as well as the release of the cycloxygenase and lipoxygenase. PAF release can also be initiated by stimulation of the complement or coagulation systems, resulting in increased pulmonary leukostasis. Stimulation of the arachidonic acid cascade by complement or other factors can affect pulmonary function. The lipoxygenase pathway results in leukotriene accumulation which can interact with white blood cells and eventually alter lung permeability. Earlier studies suggested that neutropenia may be protective in this regard, however, this has not been borne out by several clinical studies.[16] The cycloxygenase pathway results in the accumulation of both, prostacyclines and thromboxane. Clinically, thromboxanes are considered a likely stimulant of pulmonary vasoconstriction, while prostacyclines more likely cause the peripheral vasodilatation seen in these patients.[17]

To date, multiple studies have investigated the role of corticosteroids in sepsis, including death and the development of ARDS. There remains little definitive evidence that steroids are of any benefit in ameliorating the pulmonary response to sepsis.[18]

Stimulation of neutrophils by oxygen following reperfusion can result in the release of oxygen radicals.[19] These agents which include superoxide (O_2^-), peroxide (H_2O_2), and hydroxyl (OH^-) can alter basement membranes, the interstitial matrix, and neutralize antiproteases. Pulmonary changes include altered permeability and weight gain as water accumulates in the interstitial space. Antioxidants include superoxide dismutase, catalase, acetylcysteine, and vitamin E. Recent studies have demonstrated that the development of toxic oxygen radicals originally felt to be an immediate event following injury, can be delayed almost 24 hours.[20] This may present opportunities to develop clinical strategies for treatment.

Complement activation stimulated by the release of endotoxin can follow soft tissue injury and the development of conditions such as pancreatitis. Neutrophil stimulation results from release of C5a and ultimately leukocyte catalyses are released. These also can interfere with capillary permeability.

Recent studies also indicate that macrophage stimulation by eicosanoids are related to the ratio of N-6 polyunsaturated fatty acids (derived from vegetable oil) to N-3 polyunsaturated fatty acids (derived from fish oil). As this ratio increases above unity, increased eicosinoid release takes place.[21] During sepsis the administration of N-3 polyunsaturated fatty acids may modulate the entire systemic and pulmonary response. This agent will soon become available in enteral feeds.

The clinician should not approach ARDS as an isolated specific pulmonary injury requiring treatment. It is clear that neither, ventilatory support nor antibiotic therapy provide more than supportive care. Instead, pulmonary dysfunction must be considered a marker of a more involved systemic response usually to sepsis. Continued investigations into the various mediators may hold the clue to further therapy.

During an episode of sepsis or SIRS, cardiovascular function undergoes several significant alterations.[22,23] These all appeared related to the release of various cytokines and likely endotoxins. These changes include ventricular dilation and altered contractility. This results in a decrease in ejection fraction, but usually preservation of stroke volume. Simultaneously, systemic hypotension secondary to peripheral vasodilatation also develops. The reduced systemic vascular resistance no doubt aids in the maintenance of stroke volume and cardiac output. These peripheral vascular responses appear to be mediated primarily through the release of the endothelial relaxant factor, nitrous oxide.[24] At the time of initial presentation about 90 percent of septic patients have the response illustrated. Perhaps ten percent initially have a reduced cardiac output without peripheral vasodilatation.

In addition to the efforts directed at control and treatment of sepsis the clinician must also deal with the profound cardiovascular depression. Initially, efforts are directed at reversal of hypotension. Fluid infusion must increase to meet the expanded intravascular requirement secondary to the vasodilatation. The particular fluid makes little difference provided it is at least isotonic. Therefore, normal saline should take precedence over the hypotonic Ringer's lactate. However, large volumes may result in hyperchloremia and metabolic acidosis. Colloids such as Plasmanate or Hetastarch can also be utilized. While they may be more expensive, they usually require less overall volume to reach the same endpoint. Hypertonic saline infusion will also result in less volume infused, but the extra chloride can contribute to the development of a metabolic acidosis.

Despite volume expansion, fluid therapy alone may not be sufficient to reverse the shock state. When sufficient volume has been administered, as indicated by changes in central venous or pulmonary artery occlusion pressure, inotropic support may be necessary. This occurrence is consistent with the usual known alterations in contractility present during sepsis. Epinephrine usually works best to restore blood pressure and improve cardiac contractility. In septic patients dobutamine often causes vasodilatation. Dopamine is prone to increasing heart rate.

Heart rate while usually increased in septic shock can cause significant myocardial ischemia. This is particularly so in older patients with underlying coronary artery disease. These individuals have a fixed myocardial blood flow. Heart rate should be maintained at below 100/min. Diltiazem at infusion rates up to 25 mg/hr has proved beneficial at reaching such goals without altering contractility.

Hemoglobin levels should always be maintained between 10-13 gm/dL. This will ease cardiac work and will not alter microcirculatory flow. In terms of oxygen delivery, a gram of hemoglobin is the equivalent of a one liter cardiac output increase.

It has become increasingly clear that resuscitation in septic shock must be focused beyond merely blood pressure or cardiac output. In septic shock, the linkage of oxygen delivery (DO_2) to oxygen consumption (VO_2) most likely extends beyond the DO_2 levels found in the resting state.[25]

While not conclusive, several studies have now demonstrated a relationship between ultimate outcome and the level of DO_2 achieved. However, survivors have almost always achieved significantly higher DO_2 levels.[26,27] It appears there is no difference related to whether the patient alone can achieve levels in excess of 500-700 mL/min/m^2 or they require significant inotropic support. The ability to achieve such levels may reflect the still intact cellular respiratory system.

In conclusion, sepsis and SIRS involves a complicated series of interactions. Respiratory and cardiac dysfunction serve as markers of the severity of the process. Treatment can restore function, but may not necessarily alter outcome. An ability to attain threshold levels of oxygen delivery may reflect the intact state of the organism and likelihood of survival.

REFERENCES

1. American College of Chest Physicians/Society of Critical Care Medicine Consensus Conference: Definitions for sepsis and organ failure and guidelines for the use of innovative therapies in sepsis. Crit Care Med, 1992;20:864-874.
2. The Veterans Administration Systemic Sepsis Cooperative Study Group. Effect of high dose glucocorticoid therapy on mortality in patients with clinical signs of systemic sepsis. N Engl J Med, 1987;317:659-665.
3. Meyrick B: Pathology of the adult respiratory distress syndrome. Crit Care Clinics, 1986;2:405-428.
4. Brigham KL, Woolverton WC, Blake LH, et al: Increased sheep lung vascular permeability caused by pseudomonas bacteria. J Clin Investigation, 1974;54:792.
5. Suffredini AF, Fromm RE, Parker, MM, et al: The cardiovascular response of normal humans to the administration of endotoxin. N Engl J Med, 1989;321:280-287.
6. Danner RL, Elin RJ, Hosseini JM, et al: Endotoxin in human septic shock. Chest, 1991;19:169-175.
7. Ziegler EJ, Fischer CJ, Sprung, CL, et al: Treatment of gram negative bacteremia and septic shock with HA-1A human monoclonal antibody against endotoxin: A randomized double-blind, placebo controlled study. N Engl J Med, 1991;324:429-436.
8. Michie HR, Manogue KR, Spriggs DR, et al: Detection of circulating tumor necrosis factor after endotoxin administration. N Engl J Med, 1988;318:1481-1486.
9. Debets JMH, Kampmeijer R, Van der Linden MPMH, et al: Plasma tumor necrosis factor and mortality in critically ill septic patients. Crit Care Med., 1989;17:489-494.
10. Stephens KE, Ishizaka A, Larrick JW, et al: Tumor necrosis factor causes increased pulmonary permeability and edema: comparison to septic acute lung injury. Am Rev Resp Dis., 1988;137:1364.
11. Tracey JJ, Fong Y, Hesse BG: Anticachectin/TNS monoclonal antibodies prevent septic shock during lethal bacteriaemia. Nature, 1987;330:662.

12. Dinarello CA: Interleukin-1 and Interleukin-1 antagonism. Blood, 1991;8;77:1627-52.
13. Ayala A, Kisala JM, Fett JA, et al: Does endotoxin tolerance prevent the release of inflammatory monotrines (Interleukin 1, Interleukin 6, or tumor necrosis factor) during sepsis. Arch Surg, 1991;127:191-97.
14. León P, Redmond HP, Shou J, et al: Interleukin-1 and its relationship to endotoxin tolerance. Arch Surg, 1992;127:146-51.
15. Mojarad M, Hamasaki Y, Said SI: Platelet activating factor increases pulmonary microvascular permeability and induces pulmonary edema: a preliminary report. Clinical Respiratory Physiology, 1983;19:253.
16. Rinaldo JE: Medication of ARDS by leukocytes: Clinical evidence and implications for therapy. Chest, 1986;89:590-593.
17. Malik AB, Perlman MB, Cooper JA, et al: Pulmonary microvascular effects of arachidonic acid metabolites and their role in lung vascular injury. Federation Proceeding, 1985;44:36.
18. Putterman C: Use of corticosteroids in the adult respiratory distress syndrome: A clinical review. J Crit Care, 1990;5:241-251.
19. Riley PM, Schiller HJ, Bulkley GB: Pharmacologic approach to tissue injury mediated by free radicals and other reactive oxygen metabolites. Am J Surg., 1991;161:488-502.
20. Nelson K, Herndon B, Leisz G: Pulmonary effects of ischemic limb reperfusion: Evidence for a role for oxygen derived radicals. Crit Care Med., 1991:19:360-363.
21. Cerra FB: Nutrient modulation of the inflammatory and immune function. Am J Surg., 1991;261:230-234.
22. Bone RC: Gram-negative sepsis, background, clinical features, and intervention. Chest, 1991;100:802-08.
23. Jardin F, Brun-Ney D, Auvert B, et al: Sepsis related cardiogenic shock. Crit Care Med, 1990;18:1055-1060.
24. Kilbourn RB, Jubran A, Gross SS, et al: Reversal of endotoxin-mediated shock by NG-methyl-L-arginine, an inhibitor of nitric oxide synthesis. Biochem Biophys Res Commun. 1990;172:1132-1138.
25. Vormeij CG, Feenstra BWA, Adrichem WJ, et al: Independent oxygen uptake and oxygen delivery in septic and post operative patients. Chest, 1991; 99:1438-1443.
26. Hayes MA, Yaw EHS, Timmins AC, et al: Response of critically ill patients to treatment aimed at achieving supranormal oxygen delivery and consumption: Relationship to outcome. Chest, 1993;103:886-895.
27. Shoemaker WC, Appel PL, Kram HB, et al: Prospective trial of supranormal values of survivors as therapeutic goals in high risk surgical patients. Chest, 1988;94:1176-1186.

PROPHYLAXIS AND THERAPEUTIC CLINICAL TRIALS IN SEVERE SEPSIS AND SEPTIC SHOCK

Gus J. Slotman, M.D.

University of Medicine and Dentistry of New Jersey
Robert Wood Johnson Medical School at Camden
Cooper Hospital/University Medical Center
Camden, New Jersey

Mortality from severe sepsis and septic shock is thought to occur from the host response to the infection. Endogenous inflammatory mediators are released, and cause endothelial damage, increased capillary permeability, failure of vital end-organs and death. These events are depicted schematically in Figure 1. Under physiologic conditions, acute phase reactants coordinate beneficially in order to maintain homeostasis and response effectively to localized microbial infection. During overwhelming sepsis, however, diffuse mediator activation results in a discoordinated attack against normal vascular endothelium. Under these conditions, increased capillary permeability, fluid leak from the intravascular space to the interstitium and end-organ dysfunction result in mortality ranging from 30 to 80 percent, if the source of sepsis can not be eradicated.[1]

A number of recent, prospective clinical trials have been directed at improving survival from severe sepsis and septic shock. The purpose of these studies has been either to prevent the colonization overgrowth of resistant micro-organisms or to bind circulating gram negative endotoxin or to beneficially modify detrimental host responses. The results of these investigations and the clinical significance of new developments in the treatment of severe sepsis and septic shock therapy are discussed below.

ANTI-FUNGAL PROPHYLAXIS IN CRITICALLY ILL SURGICAL PATIENTS

Among critically ill patients, fungal infection has become an increasingly frequent cause of septic morbidity and mortality.[2,3] In an effort to prevent such infections, nystatin has been administered prophylactically via the gut for many year, but has prevented fungal infections among the

Critical Issues in Surgery, Edited by A. C. Cernaianu et al.
Plenum Press, New York, 1995

69

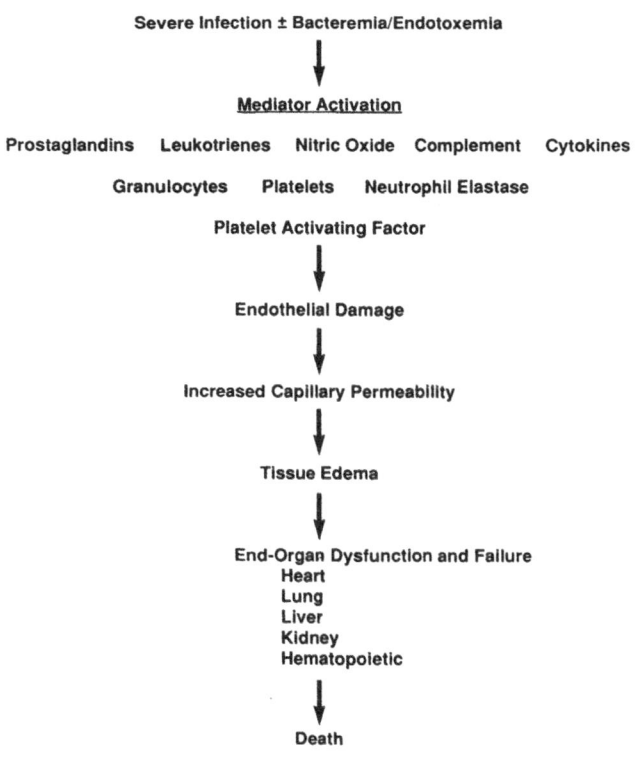

Figure 1. Systemic sepsis/septic shock pathophysiology.

critically ill only when given immediately after acute burn injury, before other risk factors for infection have become established.[4] In contrast, nystatin failures have been reported frequently in reviews of surgical patients with fungemia.[2,3]

Ketoconazole is an imidazole-based antifungal that is absorbed systemically after once-a-day enteral administration. Its systemic effects suggest that ketoconazole might prevent fungal colonization and invasive infection more effectively than the non-absorbable nystatin, which acts only within the gut lumen. Slotman et al tested this concept in a prospective, randomized, double-blind placebo controlled clinical trial in critically ill surgical patients and found that ketoconazole significantly decreased fungal colonization.[5] Invasive fungal infection was significantly decreased as well to 0 percent in the ketoconazole group, compared with 11 percent among patients receiving placebo. The antifungal effectiveness of enteral ketoconazole in preventing fungal sepsis was clinically significant, as most patients in the study had undergone gastrointestinal surgery.

Fluconazole, an azole-based, antifungal preparation which is absorbed enterally or can be given as an intravenous infusion is promising theoretically as a means of preventing fungal infections among critically ill surgical patients.[6] Its availability for parenteral administration may give fluconazole an advantage over ketoconazole in the surgical intensive care unit setting. A surgical prophylaxis clinical trial of fluconazole compared with placebo is underway.

HIGH-DOSE STEROIDS IN SYSTEMIC SEPSIS AND SEPTIC SHOCK

After animal investigations,[7] using canine and primate endotoxemia paradigms indicated that high-dose corticosteroids significantly improved survival, initial clinical studies were promising, but inconclusive.[8,9] After several dozen studies of glucocorticoid therapy in bacterial infection failed to define the role of steroid treatment conclusively,[9] four prospective, randomized, placebo controlled double-blind clinical trials were carried out during the past decade. Hoffman[10] and Sprung, et al[11] conducted pilot studies on patients with bacteremia, hypotension, and altered mental status, in which dexamethasone and methylprednisolone sodium succinate significantly reduced mortality, compared to placebo. Subsequently, however, two large studies of high-dose methylprednisolone in severe sepsis and septic shock found that high-dose steroids were without survival benefit and did not improve end-organ failure.[12,13] Recovery from secondary infection was better among patients receiving placebo than for the steroid group in the Veteran's Administrative Cooperative Study.[12] The Methylprednisolone Severe Sepsis Study Group[13] found mortality to be significantly increased among methylprednisolone patients with serum creatinine greater than 2 mg/dL, compared with placebo (58 percent vs. 29 percent, $p<0.01$). In addition, there were more deaths as a result of secondary infection with methylprednisolone.[12] Further retrospective analysis of the Methylprednisolone Severe Sepsis Study Group data indicated significant worsening of serum bilirubin and blood urea nitrogen levels with steroid treatment, compared with placebo.[14] These results of clinical trials evaluating high-dose corticosteroids in sepsis and septic shock indicate that this treatment cannot be recommended. The known adverse effects of these agents and their lack of clinical efficacy outweigh any potential good. High-dose corticosteroids, therefore, should not be administered empirically in the treatment of septic shock.

ARACHIDONIC ACID METABOLITES IN SEPSIS AND ORGAN FAILURE

Prostaglandins have been indicated as mediators of the hemodynamic derangements of systemic sepsis. Thromboxane A_2 is involved in the increased pulmonary vascular resistance, intravascular platelet aggregation and hemodynamic embarrassment of experimental,[15,16] and clinical[17,18] septic shock. Prostacyclin, which may be responsible for peripheral vasodilation in septic shock[18,19] has potential as a therapeutic agent also, because of its ability to improve hemodynamics and preserve tissue integrity.[20] Prostaglandin E_1 (PGE$_1$), physiologically similar in action to prostacyclin, may also have therapeutic potential in critical illness.[21]

Bihari and co-workers investigated exogenous intravenous prostacyclin in critically ill patients.[22] They observed hemodynamic improvement, accompanied by systemic hypotension. These results suggested that the therapeutic margin of safety of prostacyclin might not be adequate for its use in septic patients. The data did not identify a potential survival benefit for prostacyclin.

After a promising pilot study of PGE_1 in the adult respiratory distress syndrome (ARDS),[23] a multi-institutional clinical trial of PGE_1 in ARDS was carried out. PGE_1 improved hemodynamic function compared with placebo but pulmonary function and survival were not changed.[24] A subsequent evaluation of 150 patients who received either PGE_1 or placebo in ARDS revealed hemodynamic improvement, plus beneficial changes in serum bilirubin and AST blood levels and in white cell availability among patients receiving PGE_1.[25] As a single agent, prostaglandin E_1 does not change mortality in ARDS resulting from sepsis or trauma. Its beneficial biological properties, however, may allow it to become an important adjuvant tool in our therapeutic armamentarium.

Another attractive therapeutic possibility is the inhibition of detrimental prostaglandins, such as thromboxane A_2. Leeman[26] and Reines,[27] in separate studies, administered the thromboxane synthetase inhibitor dazoxiben intravenously to critically ill patients. Significant changes in systemic or pulmonary hemodynamics or in alveolar capillary gas exchange were not observed.

Ketoconazole, the imidazole-based antifungal compound, also is a specific inhibitor of thromboxane synthetase[28] and 5-lipoxygenase.[29] Investigators theorized that, as an inhibitor of these specific septic shock mediators, ketoconazole might be effective in preventing end-organ dysfunction. Seventy-one surgical intensive care unit patients at high risk for ARDS were randomized to receive either ketoconazole or placebo[30] in a prospective, double-blind clinical trial. The incidence of ARDS was decreased significantly with ketoconazole compared with placebo (6 percent vs. 31 percent, p<0.01), as were surgical intensive care unit (SICU) stay, SICU cost, and plasma thromboxane levels. The authors concluded that ketoconazole was an effective agent for preventing ARDS in critically ill patients.

ANTIENDOTOXIN ANTIBODIES IN SEPSIS

Subsequent to the sentinel study of a human antiserum to the escherichia coli J5 core lipopolysaccharide,[31] in which survival is improved with the J5 antiserum among patients with bacteremia, hypotension, and profound shock, the development of monoclonal antibody technology resulted in two perspective randomized trials of anti-endotoxin antibodies in severe sepsis and septic shock. Neither the HA1A human antibody against *Escherichia coli* J5,[32] or the E5 murine monoclonal IgM anti-endotoxin antibody[33] improved survival overall in the sepsis syndrome. Among the 200 patients with gram-negative bacteremia in the HA1A study, mortality was significantly decreased by HA1A compared with placebo (30 percent vs. 49 percent, p = 0.014). E5 patients with gram-negative sepsis who were not in shock had a lower mortality than did placebo patients for the same clinical characteristics. The failure of these two studies to improve survival from systemic sepsis overall leaves the role of antiendotoxin antibodies undefined. Further clinical trials may confirm the efficacy of antiendotoxin antibody therapy among patients with gram-negative bacteremia and shock.

CYTOKINE MODULATION IN SEPSIS

Interleukin-1 and tumor necrosis factor have been implicated as causative agents in the host response to severe sepsis.[34,35] Exogenous tumor necrosis factor,[36] and interleukin-1,[37] when administered to experimental animals, result in a shock-like state. Inhibitors of these cytokines improved survival in experimental sepsis.[38,39] These results suggested a possible therapeutic role for cytokine antagonists in septic sepsis. A phase II trial of a naturally occurring human protein interleukin-1 receptor antagonist (IL-1ra) resulted in significantly improved survival in a dose response, analytical format.[40] Subsequent Phase III multi-institutional study did not confirm this survival benefit of IL-1ra overall but suggested that IL-1 inhibition may be therapeutic in selected subgroups of septic patients.[41]

In a pilot clinical trial, Fisher and co-workers administered an anti-tumor necrosis factor monoclonal antibody to 80 patients with severe sepsis or septic shock.[42] No survival benefit was found in the principal study population, but patients with increasing circulating tumor necrosis factor concentrations at study entry may have benefitted. Further clinical trials of tumor necrosis factor are in severe sepsis and septic shock are currently being organized.

SUMMARY

Ketoconazole is an effective agent in the prophylaxis of fungal colonization and invasive fungal infection from surgical intensive care unit patients at risk. This imidazole-based antifungal, possibly due to its inhibition of thromboxane A_2 and leukotrine synthesis, is effective also in preventing ARDS in critically ill surgical patients. The lack of clinical efficacy of corticosteroids in septic shock has been demonstrated, and the potential dangers of steroids exacerbating end-organ dysfunction should be considered in planning the management therapy of critically ill patients. Antiendotoxin monoclonal antibodies may improve survival from gram-negative septic shock, but subclinical means of identifying these patients has not been developed. Promising inhibitors of interleukin-1 and tumor necrosis factor are currently being studied in prospective randomized double-blind placebo controlled clinical trials.

REFERENCES

1. Knaus WA, Sun X, Nystrom P, et al: Evaluation of definitions for sepsis. Chest 1992;101:1656-1692.
2. DeGregoria MW, Lee MWMF, Ries CA: Candida infections in patients with acute leukemia: Ineffectiveness of nystatin prophylaxis and relationship between oropharyngeal and systemic candidiasis. Cancer 1982;50:2780-2784.

3. Burchard KW, Minor LB, Slotman GJ: Fungal sepsis in surgical patients. Arch Surg 1983;118:217-221.

4. Stone HH: Studies in the pathogenesis, diagnoses and treatment of candida sepsis in children. J Pediatr Surg 1974;9:127-132.

5. Slotman GJ, Burchard KW: Ketoconazole prevents candida sepsis in critically ill patients. Arch Surg 1987;122:147-151.

6. Morrow JD: Fluconazole - A new triazole antifungal agent. Am J Med Sci 1991;302:129-132.

7. Hinshaw LB: Current concepts and future developments. Acta Chir Scand 1985;526(Supp):129-137.

8. Wilson RF, Fisher CJ: The hemodynamic effects of massive steroids in clinical shock. Surg Gynecol Obstet 1968;127:769-776.

9. Weitzmans S, Burger S: Clinical trial design and studies of corticoid steroids for bacterial infections. Ann Intern Med 1974;81:31-42.

10. Hoffman SL, Puniabi NH, Kumala S, et al: Reduction of mortality in chloramphenicol-treated severe typhoid fever by high-dose dexamethasone. N Engl J Med 1984;310:82-88.

11. Sprung CL, Caralis PV, Marcial EH, et al: The effects of high-dose corticosteroids in patients with septic shock. N Engl J Med 1984;311:1137-1143.

12. The Veterans Administration Systemic Sepsis Cooperative Study Group: Effect of high-dose glucocorticoid therapy on mortality in patients with clinical signs of systemic sepsis. N Engl J Med 1987;317:659-665.

13. Bone RC, Fisher CJ, Clemmer TP, et al: A controlled clinical trial of high-dose methylprednisolone in the treatment of severe sepsis and septic shock. N Engl J Med 1987;317:653-658.

14. Slotman GJ, Fisher CJ, Bone RC, et al: Detrimental effects of high-dose methylprednisolone sodium succinate (MPSS) on hepatic and renal function in clinical severe sepsis and septic shock. Circ Shock 1991;34:131.

15. Slotman GJ, Yellin SA, Handy JR: Thromboxane A_2 mediates hemodynamic and respiratory dysfunction in graded bacteremia. Surgery 100:214-221, 1986.

16. Huval WD, Dunham BM, Lelcuk S, et al: Thromboxane mediation of cardiovascular dysfunction following aspiration. Surgery 1983;94:259-266.

17. Hulushka PV, Reines HD, Barrow SE, et al: Elevated plasma 6-ketoprostaglandin $F_{1\alpha}$ in patients in septic shock. Crit Care Med 1985;13:451-453.

18. Slotman GJ, Burchard KW, et al: Interaction of prostaglandins, activated complement, and granulocytes in clinical sepsis and hypotension. Surgery 1986;99:744-750.

19. Slotman GJ, Quinn JV, Burhcard KW, et al: Thromboxane interaction with cardiopulmonary dysfunction ingraded bacterial sepsis. J Trauma 1984;24:803-810.

20. Slotman GJ, Machiedo GW, Casey KF, et al: Histologic and hemodynamic effects of prostacyclin and prostaglandin E1 following oleic acid infusion. Surgery 1982;92:92-100.

21. Sinclair SB, Greig PD, Lendis LM, et al: Biochemical and clinical response of fulminant viral hepatitis to administration of prostaglandin E_1: A preliminary report. J Clin Invest 1989;84:1063-1069.

22. Bihari D, Smithies M, Gimson A, et al: The effects of vasodilation with prostacyclin on oxygen delivery and uptake in critically ill patients. N Engl J Med 1987;317:397-403.

23. Holcroft JW, Vassar MJ, Weber CJ: Prostaglandin E_1 and survival in patients with the adult respiratory distress syndrome. Ann Surg 1986;203:371-378.

24. Bone RC, Slotman G, Maunder R, et al: Randomized, double-blind, multicenter study of prostaglandin E_1 in patients with adult respiratory distress syndrome. Chest 1989;96:114-119.

25. Slotman GJ, Kerstein MD, Bone RC, et al: The effects of prostaglandin E_1 on non-pulmonary organ function during clinical acute respiratory failure. J Trauma 1992;32:480-489.

26. Leeman M, Boeynaems J, Degaute J, et al: Administration of dazoxiben, a selective thromboxane synthetase inhibitor, in the adult respiratory distress syndrome. Chest 1985;87:726-730.

27. Reines HD, Halushka PV, Olanoff LW, et al: Dazoxiben in human sepsis and adult respiratory distress syndrome. Clin Pharmacol Ther 1985;37:391-395.

28. Lelcuk S, Huval WV, Valeri CR, et al: Inhibition of ischemia-induced thromboxane synthesis in man. J Trauma 1984;24:393-396.
29. Beetens JR, Loots W, Somer SY, et al: Ketoconazole inhibits the biosynthesis of leukotrines in vitro and in vivo. Biochem Pharmacol 1986;35:883-891.
30. Slotman GJ, Burchard KW, D'Arezzo A, et al: Ketoconazole prevents acute respiratory failure in critically ill surgical patients. J Trauma 1988;28:648-654.
31. Ziegler EJ, McCuthcan A, Fierer J, et al: Treatment of negative bacteremia and shock with human antiserum to a mutan Escherichia coli. N Engl J Med 1982;307:1225-1230.
32. Ziegler EJ, Fisher CJ, Sprung CL, et al: Treatment of gram-negative bacteremia and septic shock with HA-1A human monoclonal antibody against endotoxin. N Engl J Med 1991;324:429-436.
33. Greenman RL, Schein RMH, Martin MA, et al: A controlled clinical trial of E5 murine monoclonal IgM antibody to endotoxin in the treatment of gram-negative sepsis. JAMA 1991;266:1097-1102.
34. Roten R, Markert M, Feihl F, et al: Plasma levels of tumor necrosis factor in the adult respiratory distress syndrome. Am Rev Respir Dis 1991;143:590-592.
35. Girardin E, Grau GE, Dayer JM et al: Tumor necrosis factor and interleukin-1 in the serum of children with severe infectious purpura. N Engl J Med 1988;319:397-400.
36. Schirmer WJ, Schirmer JM, Fry DE: Recombinant human tumor necrosis factor produces hemodynamic changes characteristic of sepsis and endotoxemia. Arch Surg 1989;124:445-448.
37. Dinarello Ca, Okusawa S, Gelfand JA: Interleukin-1 induces a shock-like state in rabbits: Synergism with tumor necrosis factor and the effect of cyclo-oxygenase inhibition. In: molecular and cellular mechanisms of septic shock. Alan R Liss, Inc., 1989:243-263.
38. Ohlsson K, Bjork P, Bergeinfeldt M, et al: An interleukin-1 receptor antagonist reduces mortality from endotoxic shock. Nature 1990;348:550-552.
39. Opal SM, Cross AS, Kelly NM, et al: Efficacy of a monoclonal antibody directed against tumor necrosis factor in protecting neutropenic rats from lethal infection with pseudomonas aeruginosa. J Infect Dis 1990;161:1148-1152.
40. Fisher CJ, Slotman GJ, Opal SM, et al: Interleukin-1 receptor antagonist (IL-1ra) reduces mortality in patients with sepsis syndrome. American College of Chest Physicians, November 7, 1991 (Abstract).
41. Fisher CJ, Dhainaut JF, Pribble JP, and the IL-1ra Phase III Sepsis Syndrome Study Group: A study to evaluate the safety and efficacy of human recombinant interleukin-1 receptor antagonist in the treatment of patients with sepsis. syndrome. 13th International Symposium on Intensive Care and Emergency Medicine. Brussels, Belgium, March, 1993.
42. Fisher CJ JR, Opal SM, Dhainaut JF, et al: Influence of an anti-tumor necrosis factor monoclonal antibody on cytokine levels in patients with sepsis. Crit Care Med 1993;21(3):318-327.

PHARMACOLOGIC MANAGEMENT OF POSTOPERATIVE INFECTIONS

Jacqueline D. Sutton, Pharm.D.

University of Medicine and Dentistry of New Jersey
Robert Wood Johnson Medical School
Cooper Hospital/University Medical Center
Camden, New Jersey

Although the incidence of postoperative infections is controversial, approximately 30 percent of hospitalized surgical patients develop infections accounting for almost 70 percent of nosocomial infections. Thus, *antibiotic* therapy including antibacterials, antivirals, antifungals is an essential consideration. For effective antibiotic therapy, several factors must be determined including patient evaluation, antibiotic selection (empiric vs. specific vs. prophylaxis) and patient monitoring while on therapy.

SURGICAL PROPHYLAXIS

The use of prophylactic antibiotics are useful, particularly, to decrease the incidence of wound infections. Prophylaxis is indicated for high infection rate procedures and prosthesis implantation for minimizing infections around the wound or internal manipulation sites. However, antibiotic use is not without risks, i.e., toxicity, allergy, resistance, and superinfection. Thus, benefits should balance the associated risks. Several factors should be considered for prophylactic antibiotic selection.

Types of Infection

The potential type of infecting organism needs to be determined. *Staphylococcus* infections are still the single most common gram negative infections, however, *E. coli, Pseudomonas, Enterobacter,* and *Proteus* collectively increased greater than *Staphylococcus* alone.

Critical Issues in Surgery, Edited by A. C. Cernaianu et al.
Plenum Press, New York, 1995

Table 1. Wound Classification by Surgical
Procedure

Clean	
Cardiac ·	Orthopedic
Neurosurgery	Vascular
Ocular	
Clean-Contaminated	
Appendectomy	Gastric
Biliary	Head-neck
Cesarean section	Hysterectomy
Colorectal	Urologic
Dirty	
Ruptured viscus	
Traumatic wound	

Risk Factors

Risk factors for postoperative infections correlate with the use of antibiotics. Exogenous or endogenous sources of contamination should be considered. Exogenous contaminants may be minimal if good operating room procedures/techniques are maintained. Endogenous contamination depends on the area of incision as well as the preoperative use of antiseptics such as chlorhexidine. Awareness of potential resistance in different populations is necessary since elderly and infants, obese, malnourished, and diabetics patients are prone to more colonization with resistant organisms. Classification of wounds is helpful in the determination of the risk of infection. Contaminated and dirty procedures have a significantly higher infection rate than clean procedures.

Surgical Procedures

Clean procedures may potentially become contaminated through the surgical incision with *Staphylococci*. Antiseptic coverage should be directed to these organisms. Clean-contaminated procedures require gram negative organism coverage and anaerobic coverage depending on the objective. Dirty procedures require prophylactic coverage for gram positive and gram negative and additional postoperative anaerobic coverage extended for approximately 7 days.

Prevention

Infection control and preventative measures are essential mechanisms to minimize and/or eliminate infections. Additionally, the use of appropriate prophylactic antimicrobials in recommended procedures with proper timing and duration is helpful. One hour preoperative administration of a single dose of antibiotic may ensure antibiotic presence before bacteria is introduced and may provide adequate tissue concentration. The infection rates may increase if the antibiotic is administered intraoperatively only. In the case of prolonged procedures or extensive blood loss, a second intraop-

Table 2. Procedures Requiring Prophylaxis for Bacterial
Endocarditis

Cardiac
Valve repair/replacement
Previous bacterial endocarditis
Congenital cardiac defects
Hypertrophic cardiomyopathy
Other Surgical Procedures
Dental
Tonsillectomy/adenoidectomy
Rigid bronchoscopy
Esophageal varice sclerotherapy/dilatation
Cholecystectomy
Cystoscopy
Urethral dilatation, catheterization and/or urinary tract surgery
Prostatic surgery
Vaginal hysterectomy/delivery in presence of infection
Incision and drainage of infected tissue

erative dose may be needed. Postoperative doses are unnecessary, especially since longer half-life agents are generally used. Exceptions include dirty wounds or placement of chest tube post cardiothoracic surgery. Prophylaxis for bacterial endocarditis is necessary in specific population undergoing different surgical procedures. Table 2 reviews the current recommendations by the American Heart Association for procedures where prevention of bacterial endocarditis is necessary.

Table 3a presents different antibiotic regimens for prophylaxis of bacterial endocarditis during dental, oral and upper respiratory tract procedures. Table 3b presents specific antibiotic regimens for prophylaxis of bacterial endocarditis during genitourinary and gastrointestinal procedures.

It is important to stress that prophylactic regimens may not protect certain patients from developing infections.

PATIENT EVALUATION

Clinical assessment may assist in the process of antibiotic selection. Absence or presence of fever, shaking chills, nonspecific symptoms, specific symptoms at the infection site, exudates and/or altered white blood cell count should be considered in the empiric diagnosis of infection. Fever may be due to noninfectious reasons such as drug administration, non-dose related drug hypersensitivity, pharmacologic action of drugs or altered thermoregulation as in the case of tricyclic antidepressants or antipsychotics. Moreover, there are predisposing factors to opportunistic infections such as immunosuppression, altered normal flora, or special conditions such as in the case of intravenous drug abusers and/or the presence of indwelling, i.v. and urinary catheters.

Table 3a. Specific Antibiotic Regimens for Prophylaxis of Bacterial Endocarditis During Dental, Oral, and Upper Respiratory Tract Procedures

	1-2 hours preprocedure	6 hours postprocedure
Standard regimen		
Adult	amoxicillin 3.0 g	1.5 g po
Pediatric*	amoxicillin 50 mg/kg	25 mg/kg po
Penicillin allergic		
Adult	erythromycin steareate 1.0 g	500 mg po
	800 mg ethylsuccinate	400 mg po
Pediatric*	20 mg/kg	10 mg/kg po
Adult	clindamycin 300 mg	150 mg po
Pediatric*	clindamycin 10 mg/kg	5 mg/kg po
Unable to take oral medications		
Adult	ampicillin 2.0 g	1.0 g im/iv
		(or amoxicillin 1.5 g po)
Pediatric*	ampicillin 50 mg/kg	25 mg/kg im/iv
		(or amoxicillin 25 mg/kg po)
Adult	clindamycin 300 mg	150 mg iv/po
Pediatric*	clindamycin 10 mg/kg	5 mg/kg iv/po
High risk, penicillin allergic		
Adult	vancomycin 1.0 g iv	no repeat dose
Pediatric*	vancomycin 20 mg/kg iv	no repeat dose

*Total pediatric dose should not exceed total adult dose.

Table 3b. Specific Antibiotic Regimens for Prophylaxis of Bacterial Endocarditis During Genitourinary and Gastrointestinal Procedures

	Preprocedure	Postprocedure
Standard regimen		
Adult	ampicillin 2.0 g iv/im +	amoxicillin 1.5 g po
	gentamicin 1.5 mg/kg iv/im	(or repeat iv/im regimen 8 hr after first dose)
Pediatric*	ampicillin 50 mg/kg iv/im +	amoxicillin 25 mg/kg po
	gentamicin 2.0 mg/kg iv/im	(or repeat iv/im regimen 8 hr after first dose)
Penicillin allergic		
Adult	vancomycin 1.0 g iv +	may be repeated
	gentamicin 1.5 mg/kg iv/im	8 hrs
Pediatric*	vancomycin 20 mg/kg iv +	may be repeated
	gentamicin 2.0 mg/kg iv/im	8 hrs
Low risk		
Adult	amoxicillin 3.0 g	1.5 g po
Pediatric*	amoxicillin 50 mg/kg	25 mg/kg

* Total pediatric dose should not exceed total adult dose.

Table 4. Site of Infection

Site	Pathogen
Skin	*Staph. aureus, epidermidis*
	S. pyogenes
Lung	*S. pneumoniae*
	H. influenzae
	Klebsiella pneumonia
	Mycoplasma
Gastrointestinal tract	*E. Coli*
	Klebsiella
	Enterococci (S. faecalis)
	B. fragilis
	Clostridium
Urinary tract	*E. Coli*
	Klebsiella
	Proteus
	Pseudomonas
	Serratia

APPROPRIATE ANTIBIOTIC SELECTION

The specific site of infection with its likelihood for bacterial pathogens, i.e., aerobe or anaerobe, may also help in the empiric selection of antibiotics (Table 4).

A summary of the most common pathogens encountered in postoperative infections is listed in Table 5. To actually isolate and identify the organism, several steps are necessary, including the collection of a sample *before* antibiotic initiation, review of gram stains or smears, and review of sensitivity information for exact antibiotic selection.

Specific patient characteristics may determine the most appropriate antibiotic selection. Primarily, consideration should be given to allergy

Table 5. Infectious Bacteria Classification

Aerobes	
Gram-positive cocci	*Pneumococcus, Enterococcus, S. viridans*
	Staph. aureus, Staph. epidermidis
Gram-positive bacilli	*Corynebacterium, Listeria, Clostridium*
Gram-negative cocci	*N. gonorrhoeae, N. meningitidis, Moraxella species, Branhamella catarrhalis*
Gram-negative bacilli	*E. Coli, Enterobacter, Klebsiella, Proteus, Serratia, Salmonella, Pseudomonas, Campylobacter, H. influenzae, Legionella*
Anaerobes	
Gram-positive cocci	*Peptococcus, Peptostreptococcus*
Gram-positive bacilli	*Clostridium*
Gram-negative bacilli	*B. fragilis, B. melaninogenicus*

Table 6. Spectrum of Coverage

	Vanc	Clind	Ery	Ags	Tmp/Smx	Tcn	Chloro	Imip	Metr
Gram-positive aerobes									
Staph. aureus	X	X	X		X	X	X	X	
Staph. aureus[a]	X	X			X			X	
Staph. epidermidis	X							X	
B. hemolytic Strep	X		X						
S. pneumoniae	X	X	X		X	X	X	X	
S. faecalis	X							X	
Gram-positive anaerobes									
Peptostreptococci		X					X	X	X
Clostridium		X	X					X	X
Gram-negative aerobes									
E. Coli				X	X	X	X	X	
Klebsiella				X	X		X	X	
H. influenzae				X	X	X	X	X	
Proteus indole-positive				X	X		X	X	
Proteus indole-negative				X				X	
N. gonorrheae			X		X	X		X	
Enterobacter				X				X	
Providencia				X				X	
Citrobacter				X				X	
Serratia				X				X	
Pseudomonas sp.				X				X[b]	
Gram-negative anaerobes									
B. fragilis		X						X	X

Vanc = Vancomycin; Clind = Clindamycin; Ery = Erythromycin; Ags = Aminoglycosides; Tmp/Smx = Trimethoprim/sulfamethoxazole; Tcn = Tetracycline; Chloro = Chloramphenicol; Imip = Imipenem; Metr = Metronidazole.
[a]penicillinase producing; Aztreonam—similar spectrum to aminoglycosides.
[b]not active against Pseudomonas maltophilia.

history, patient's age, organ system impairment, immune competency, concomitant diseases and genetic conditions such as glucose 6-phosphate dehydrogenase deficiency. The competency of the immune system is of utmost importance, since different bactericidal regimens and agents specific against more resistant pathogens are necessary in the presence of an incompetent immune system.

Finally, consideration pertaining to the drug is important in the selection process. The ideal agent would be narrow spectrum, bactericidal with minimal potential resistance and/or toxicity, easily administered and cost efficient.

Additional considerations require knowledge of the spectrum of coverage (Tables 6), as well as the antibiotic effect on bacteria, i.e., bactericidal vs. static perspectives (Table 7). In addition, the pharmacokinetics and pharmacodynamics of each drug as well as its toxicity, cost and the usefulness of combination therapy should be considered. Combination

Table 7. Bactericidal and Bacteriostatic Antibacterial Agents

Bactericidal	Bacteriostatic
Aminoglycosides	Chloramphenicol (low conc.)
Aztreonam	Erythromycin
Cephalosporins	Sulfonamides
Chloramphenicol (high conc.)	Tetracycline
Fluoroquinolones	Trimethoprim
Imipenem/cilastatin	
Penicillins	
Trimethoprim/sulfamethoxazole	
Vancomycin	

therapy allows broad coverage, synergy, prevention of resistance, and decreased adverse effects with minimal antagonism.

SPECIFIC ANTI-INFECTIVE AGENTS

Anti-infective agents include antibacterials, antifungals and antivirals. Each class of agents provides coverage of organisms based on specific mechanisms of action, pharmacokinetics and adverse effect profiles.

Antibacterials

The overall mechanisms of action include inhibition of bacterial cell wall synthesis, bacterial membrane function, bacterial protein or nucleic acid synthesis.

Based on spectrum of coverage, penicillins (Table 8a) are classified as natural, penicillinase-resistant, aminopenicillins or antipseudomonal penicillins. Table 8b outlines the penicillin spectrum.

Similarly, cephalosporins (Table 9) are classified as first, second or third generation with increasing gram negative coverage. Selected agents, such as cefoxitin and cefotetan, can provide anaerobic coverage for *B. fragilis* in addition to second generation spectrum.

Aminoglycosides (i.e., gentamicin) and monobactams (i.e., aztreonam) have primarily gram negative coverage. Usually, these agents are used in combination with another agent covering gram positive or extending gram negative coverage for synergy.

Carbapenems such as imipenem/cilastatin provide broad gram positive and gram negative aerobic and anaerobic coverage.

Macrolides, including azithromycin, clarithromycin, erythromycin, are primarily intended for gram positive coverage. Increased coverage may be achieved with newer agents which have slightly less gastrointestinal side effects. Fluoroquinolones such as ciprofloxacin and ofloxacin are new broad spectrum gram positive and gram negative agents lacking good anaerobic and *streptococcal/enterococcal* coverage.

Intravenous vancomycin still remains almost 100 percent effective against systemic infections with gram positive *staphylococcus* and *streptococcus* and *C. difficile* diarrhea (oral only).

Table 8a. Types of Penicillin

Natural Penicillins	Penicillin G (po,im,iv)
	Penicillin V (po)
Penicillinase Resistant Methicillin (im,iv)	
(β-lactamase)	Nafcillin (po,im,iv)
	Oxacillin (po,im,iv)
	Cloxacillin (po)
	Dicloxacillin (po)
Aminopenicillins	Ampicillin (po,im,iv)
	Amoxicillin (po)
Antipseudomonal	Carbenicillin (po)
	Ticarcillin (im,iv)
	Mezlocillin (im,iv)
	Piperacillin (im,iv)

Table 8b. Penicillin Spectrum

	Natural	Penicillinase Resistant	Amino-Penicillin	Antipseudomonal Penicillin
Gram-positive aerobes				
Staph. aureus	X	X	X	X
Staph. aureus[a]		X		
Staph. epidermidis		X		
B. hemolytic Strep	X	X	X	X
S. pneumoniae	X	X	X	X
Enterococci	X[b]	X[b]	X[b]	X[b]
Gram-positive anaerobes				
Peptostreptococci	X	X		X
Clostridium	X	X	X	X
Gram-negative aerobes				
E. Coli			X	X
Klebsiella				
H. influenzae			X	X
Proteus indole-positive			X	X
Proteus indole-negative				X
N. gonorrheae	X		X	X
N. meningitidis	X		X	X
Enterobacter				X
Providencia				X
Citrobacter				X
Serratia				X
Pseudomonas sp.				X
Gram-negative anaerobes				
B. fragilis				X[c]

[a] in combination with an aminoglycoside
[b] high dose -> 65% coverage
[c] penicillinase producing

Table 9. Cephalosporin Spectrum

First Generation	(cefazolin, cephalexin, cephalothin)
Gram-positive[a]	*S. pneumoniae*
	Staph. aureus, epidermidis
Gram-negative	*E. Coli*
	H. influenzae
	Klebsiella
	Proteus (indole-negative)
Second Generation	(cefaclor, cefamandole[b], cefonicid, cefotetan[b], cefoxitin, cefuroxime)
Gram-positive[a]	Same as first generation
	Anaerobic streptococci (i.e. S. pyogenes)
Gram-negative	Same as first generation
	Proteus indole positive
	N. gonorrheae
	Enterobacter
	B. fragilis
Third Generation[c,d]	(cefixime, cefoperazone[b], cefotaxime, ceftazidime, ceftizoxime, ceftriaxone)
Gram-positive	Same as 1st and 2nd generation but less active
Gram-negative	Same as 1st and 2nd generation; more activity at lower MIC
	Providencia
	Citrobacter
	Serratia
	Pseudomonas aeruginosa (ceftazidime > cefoperazone)

[a]No coverage for enterococci.
[b]Contains MTT side chain.
[c]No effect on methicillin resistant *Staph. aureus*, no fungal coverage.
[d]Third generation efficacy against *Staph. aureus*: cefotaxime, ceftizoxime, ceftriaxone > cefoperazone > ceftazidime; MIC = minimum inhibitory concentration.

Gram negative anaerobic infections can be effectively controlled by metronidazole and clindamycin administration.

All of these agents are options for treatment of bacterial infections, although most routine postoperative infections should not require additional agents beyond designated prophylaxis.

Antifungals

Antifungals such as amphotericin B, flucytosine, fluconazole, ketoconazole and itraconazole act by fungal cell membrane binding. These agents are effective prophylactically or as treatment agents against most common fungi. Some drugs may provide greater efficacy against resistant fungi (flucytosine, amphotericin plus flucytosine).

Antivirals

Antivirals such as acyclovir, foscarnet/ganciclovir inhibit viral DNA synthesis for effective control of herpes simplex virus (HSV) and cytomegalovirus (CMV), respectively. However, the use of these agents is usually not warranted in routine postoperative infections.

ANTIBIOTIC MONITORING

Following initiation of therapy, patients should be monitored for efficacy. Antibiotic regimens should be evaluated to determine if most likely or documented pathogens are covered. Culture and sensitivity data should determine adequate dosing and appropriate achievement of serum level. Pharmacokinetic parameters would allow dose adjustment based on serum levels and/or elimination rates to minimize adverse reactions. Individual agents should be considered for potential adverse effect and drug interactions.

Adverse Effects

Gastrointestinal symptoms such as nausea, vomiting and diarrhea resulting from superinfection with *C. difficile* are common especially with broad spectrum agents. Hematologic effects with agents such as chloramphenicol, both dose related, and idiosyncratic have been reported. Neurologic effects with high dose penicillins and imipenem warrant appropriate dosage adjustments. Renal complications such as interstitial nephritis with methicillin and increased serum creatinine with aminoglycosides or amphotericin B require additional monitoring.

Drug Interactions

Several agents must be monitored for altered pharmacologic effect or adverse effect due to significant drug interactions. For example, simultaneous administration of probenecid may increase serum levels of drugs eliminated by the renal system. Selected cephalosporins with a methylthiotetrazole (MTT) side-chain may produce hypoprothrombinemia and will potentially interact with alcohol, producing a disulfiram-like reaction. Concurrent metronidazole and alcohol administration may also result in a disulfiram-like reaction which may extend up to several days following discontinuation of therapy. Oral fluoroquinolones have decreased absorption in the presence of antacid. Moreover, aminoglycosides are inactivated by antipseudomonal penicillins and may potentially increase nephrotoxicity in the presence of agents having a similar toxic profile.

CONCLUSION

Infection control is an important step in the patient's postoperative management. With an appropriate prophylactic regimen, treatment is generally not necessary. If therapy begins, patient's evaluation, specific antibiotic selection, and appropriate monitoring based on culture and sensitivity data as well as clinical response will determine successful management.

SUGGESTED READING

Antimicrobial prophylaxis in surgery. The Medical Letter on Drugs Ther 1993;35:91.
The choice of antibacterial drugs. The Medical Letter on Drugs Ther 1994;36:53-60.

ASHP Commission on Therapeutics. ASHP therapeutic guidelines on nonsurgical antimicrobial prophylaxis. Clin Pharm 1990; 9:423-45.

Craig CR, Stitzel RE (Eds): Modern Pharmacology, 2nd ed. Boston, Little, Brown & Company; 1986.

DiPiro JT, Cheung RPF, Bowden TA, Mansberger JA: Single dose systemic prophylaxis of surgical wound infections. Am J Surg 1986;152:552-9.

DiPiro JT, Talbert RL, et al (Eds): Pharmacotherapy: A Pathophysiologic Approach, 2nd ed. New York, NY, Elsevier; 1992.

Evans WE, Schentag JJ, Jusko WJ: Applied Pharmacokinetics: Principles of Therapeutic Drug Monitoring, 2nd ed. Spokane, Washington, Applied Therapeutics Inc; 1986

Gilbert DN, Gerberding JL, Sandy NA: Guide to Antimicrobial Therapy, Sanford JP (Ed) Dallas, TX, Antimicrobial Therapy, Inc; 1993.

Guglielmo BJ, Hohn DC, Koo PJ, et al: Antibiotic prophylaxis in surgical procedures: a critical analysis of the literature. Arch Surg 1983;118:943-55.

Herfindal ET, Gourley DR, Hart LL (Eds): Clinical Pharmacy and Therapeutics, 5th ed. Baltimore, MD, Williams & Wilkins; 1992.

Kaiser AB: Antimicrobial prophylaxis in surgery. N Engl J Med 1986; 315:1129-38.

Rowland M, Tozer TN: Clinical Pharmacokinetics, 2nd ed. Philadelphia, Lea & Febiger; 1989.

Spector R: Scientific Basis of Clinical Pharmacology: Principles & Examples. Boston, Little, Brown & Company; 1986.

Sutton JD, Thalken DW, Powell MC: Nurses' IV Drug Manual. Norwalk, CT, Appleton & Lange; 1993.

Winter ME: Basic Clinical Pharmacokinetics, 2nd ed. Spokane, Washington, Applied Therapeutics Inc; 1991.

THE RESUSCITATION GAME

Mary McCarthy, M.D.

Wright State University
Miami Valley Hospital
Dayton, Ohio

RESUSCITATION OF THE TRAUMA PATIENT

You Bet Your Life

The basic principles of resuscitation of the trauma patient are well-recognized. Evaluation and management of the multiply-injured patient should proceed along the guidelines provided in the American College of Surgeons Advanced Trauma Life Support Course[1] listed in Table 1.

There are, however, several areas of controversy in the resuscitation of the trauma patient. This chapter will focus on recent research in prehospital, and critical care resuscitation, with emphasis on patients with multiple system organ failure.

PREHOSPITAL RESUSCITATION

The $64,000 Question

There is considerable debate over whether trauma patients should be resuscitated *at all* in the prehospital setting. This debate revolves around the question of "uncontrolled hemorrhage." Attempted resuscitation was unsuccessful in animal models (rats with tail amputation) with uncontrolled hemorrhage.[2] An increase in blood pressure in this circumstance may actually result in *increased* blood loss, and higher mortality. Two recent studies on the use of MAST trousers in the prehospital setting present opposing viewpoints on this issue. The first, a prospective, randomized study in 911 patients in the Houston Emergency Medical System (EMS) found an adverse effect on outcome of MAST application in patients with penetrating cardiac and thoracic vascular injury (mortality 31 percent MAST, 21 percent no-MAST, $p=0.05$).[3] In a retrospective database review of severely hypotensive trauma patients (BP < 50 mmHg) in the New York City

Critical Issues in Surgery, Edited by A. C. Cernaianu et al.
Plenum Press, New York, 1995

89

Table 1. Initial Assessment

1. Preparation
2. Triage
3. Primary Survey
   A-Airway
   B-Breathing
   C-Circulation
   D-Disability
   E-Exposure
4. Resuscitation
5. Secondary Survey
6. Postresuscitation monitoring and re-evaluation
7. Definitive Care

EMS System, an improvement in survival occurred despite an average scene time 4.7 minutes longer in the MAST patients.[4]

The impact of alternative resuscitation fluids is another area of active research. New information is emerging as a result of a better understanding of the molecular mechanisms operating in shock and resuscitation. Hemorrhagic shock can be separated into three phases which are listed in Table 2.[5]

During the first phase of hemorrhagic shock, there is a relocation of fluid into the intravascular space. The release of humoral and nervous system factors results in a contraction of the interstitial space matrix, and increased exclusion of albumin, with relocation of this protein to the plasma volume and enhancement of the plasma oncotic pressure. These changes likely occur in response to cytokine release. Knowledge of these changes allows adaptation of the resuscitation regimen to the phase of the response. During the treatment of early hypovolemic shock, colloid supplementation has been proposed as a means of reducing the amount of fluid lost from the plasma volume. However, compensatory mechanisms are already operative.

In phase II, there is obligatory extravascular sequestration of fluid. Reduced albumin exclusion results in alterations in the interstitial matrix and reexpansion to greater than normal degrees occurs.[6] A reduction in the plasma colloid oncotic pressure occurs independently. A portion of "third space" losses is intracellular accumulation, caused by a decrease in sodium-potassium ATPase pump activity. Attempts to force a diuresis through the use of colloid supplementation will only aggravate the plasma volume deficit, and result in organ system dysfunction.

During phase III, mobilization of fluid to the plasma volume occurs, with a normalization of cellular membrane potential, reactivation of the sodium pump and simultaneous contraction of the interstitial space.

Table 2. Phases of Hemorrhagic Shock

Phase I	Period of active bleeding, from injury to cessation of bleeding
Phase II	Extravascular fluid sequestration, from cessation of bleeding to point of maximal weight gain
Phase III	Intravascular refilling and diuresis, from maximal weight gain to maximal weight loss

Attempts to normalize fluid dynamics with the administration of colloid presupposes a simplistic model of capillary permeability, hydrostatic and oncotic pressures. Actually, in response to albumin supplementation, there is an increase in renal plasma flow, with a seemingly paradoxical fall in glomerular filtration rate (GFR), sodium clearance, and urine output. Increase in the osmotic and oncotic forces in the glomerular tuft, and alterations in the medullary gradient are responsible. Thus, colloid administration compounds the problems of resuscitation during this phase.

Prehospital fluid resuscitation with hypertonic saline (HS) provides another fertile area for research. This solution has been used in small volumes (250 mL 7.5 percent NaCl) to restore normal arterial blood pressure.[7] Those patients treated with HS were more effectively resuscitated and overall survival was higher.[8] Direct hemodynamic effects of HS may contribute to this effect. There is a direct vasodilation of arteriolar smooth muscle, and a decrease in vasoconstrictive hormones associated with volume expansion.[9] The combined effect of hemodilution and a reduction in capillary endothelial cell swelling also contributes to a decrease in microvascular resistance. Urine output increases dramatically after HS resuscitation, by promoting natriuresis, restoring renal blood flow and reducing renal tubular cell swelling. However, the addition of dextran 70 to this resuscitation regimen did not result in further improvement in outcome in patients with transport times of less than 30 minutes.[10] In addition, administration of HS in head-injured patients may improve outcome.[11] Hypertonic resuscitation may result in a shrinkage of uninjured glial and neuronal elements, thus offsetting the increases caused by the obligatory swelling of injured brain. A consequent reduction in intracranial pressure and improvement in cerebral blood flow result.

In the early phase of trauma patient resuscitation, the role of emergency thoracotomy with aortic cross-clamping is another area of investigation. Salvage of patients with blunt multiple trauma is exceedingly rare, therefore aggressive resuscitation of a patient in greater than 5 minutes of asystole is seldom justified.[12] A patient with a penetrating chest injury, especially with cardiac tamponade, will occasionally survive, therefore a longer duration of asystole is accepted (15 minutes) before resuscitation is terminated. The risk of blood exposure in these circumstances is considerable. Appropriate guidelines for the application of such aggressive resuscitative measures should be developed after evaluation of trauma center resources and results.

CRITICAL CARE RESUSCITATION

Jeopardy

Once the trauma patient has survived the initial resuscitation, the second phase of hemorrhagic shock supervenes. This phase is characterized by massive extravascular fluid sequestration. Invasive hemodynamic monitoring is indicated throughout this phase. Recent discussion has focused on the question of "adequate" resuscitation.[13] Shoemaker and his colleagues[14] have advocated resuscitation of patients to supranormal values of oxygen delivery (>650 mL/min/m^2) and consumption (>170 mL/min/m^2).

Attainment of these goals was associated with improved survival and decreased morbidity in the severely traumatized patient. However, the correlation between oxygen delivery (DO_2) and consumption (VO_2) may be related to a mathematical coupling rather than a pathologic dependence of consumption on supply.[15]

The central issue is adequacy of tissue perfusion. In addition to the global methods of measuring DO_2 and supply, newer methods are under investigation. Monitoring of tissue oxygenation may include the measurement of gastric mucosal pH, assay of the metabolites of adenine nucleotides, 31-phosphorus magnetic resonance spectroscopy, arterial lactate levels, and percutaneous fiberoptic probes with fluorescence.[16]

Inadequate resuscitation may result in translocation of bacteria and their intestinal by-products. Translocation to the mesenteric lymph nodes appeared to be uncommon in acutely injured patients,[17] however, this did not preclude the possibility that in later phases of injury, or with gastrointestinal mucosal injury, translocation by the classic route might result. In another study from Denver General Hospital, portal venous sampling through an indwelling catheter was performed in the early postoperative period.[18] Assays for gut-derived organisms, endotoxin, or cytokines were virtually identical in patients with and without organ failure.

Initiation of enteral feeding within 24 hours has been shown to maintain the integrity of the intestinal lining and inferentially to be useful in reducing the incidence of translocation.[19] Placement of feeding tubes into the upper small bowel and administration of various enteral formulas has largely replaced total parenteral nutrition as the primary mode of metabolic support. Research in this area has focused on a *nutritional prescription*, modifying formulas with the addition of specialized amino acids (arginine, glutamine), and immune system modulators (RNA, omega-6 fatty acids).[20]

MULTIPLE SYSTEM ORGAN FAILURE

Truth or Consequences

Multiple System Organ Failure (MSOF) is a syndrome which may be the final common pathway for critical illness complicated by continuing inflammation, persistent infection, severe multisystem trauma, and organ transplantation complications. The mortality is proportional to the number of organ systems failing, i.e., one organ 30 percent; two organs 60 percent; three organs 85 percent. The temporal sequence of organ system dysfunction is also remarkably consistent across the various etiologies of MSOF, with the usual pattern being lung, liver, kidneys, coagulation, and the gastrointestinal tract.[21]

MSOF is characterized by a release of systemic mediators, including cytokines, neuropeptides, and complement. Immune system activation with cell-cell interactions and toxicity occurs, and vascular endothelial damage with tissue hypoxia and ischemia results. The inflammatory mediators include interleukins, leukotrienes, prostaglandins, tumor necrosis factor, interferon, complement, proteases, and other factors which have been described in other chapters of this work. Under normal circumstances, biologic regulation of the release of these factors occurs. In MSOF the autoregulation may be disturbed. Interventional strategies employing the use of mediator blockade have been attempted, as well as use of protective factors to minimize the impact of this biological storm.

Appropriate patient care should reduce the potential for the development of MSOF. The key factors in patient care as described by Baue and Faist[22] include: 1) improving microcirculation to decrease ischemia-reperfusion injury; 2) control of tissue injury by early definitive operation; 3) debridement of necrotic tissue; 4) promoting improved oxygen transport; 5) supporting metabolism and the gut; 6) maintaining host defenses through immunomodulation, judicious use of antibiotics, and wound care, and 7) treating infection.

REFERENCES

1. Alexander RH, Proctor HJ, editors: Advanced Trauma Life Support Program for Physicians 5th ed. American College of Surgeons, Chicago, IL, 1993.
2. Peitzman A: Resuscitation of uncontrolled hemorrhage. Presentation: Eastern Association for the Surgery of Trauma (EAST), January 1994.
3. Mattox KL, Bicknell W, Pepe PE: Prospective MAST study in 911 patients. J Trauma 1989;29:1104-1112.
4. Cayten CG, Berendt BM, Byrne DW: A study of pneumatic antishock garments in severely hypotensive trauma patients. J Trauma 1993;34:728-735.
5. Geller ER, editor: Shock and Resuscitation, Chapter 5. McGraw-Hill, Inc., New York, 1993.
6. Lucas CE, Ledgerwood AM, Rachwal WJ, et al: Colloid oncotic pressure and body water dynamics in septic and injured patients. J Trauma 1991;31:927-933.
7. Vassar MJ, Perry CA, Holcroft JW: Prehospital resuscitation of hypotensive trauma patients with 7.5% NCCl versus 7.5% NcCl with added dextran: A controlled trial. J Trauma 1993;34:622-633.
8. Holcroft JW, Vassar MJ, Turner JE, et al: 3% NCCl and 7.5% NaCl/dextran 70 in the resuscitation of severely injured patients. Ann Surg 1987;206;279-288.
9. Halvorsen L, Blaisdell FW, Holcroft JW: Recent Advances in Prehospital Fluid Resuscitation: Hypertonic Saline. Adv Trauma, Vol. 5, Maull KI, Cleveland HC, Strauch GO, Wolfert CC (editors): Mosby, St. Louis., 1990.
10. Vassar JF, Fischer RP, O'Brien PE, et al: A multicenter trial for resuscitation of injured patients with 7.5% sodium chloride. Arch Surg 1993;128:1003-1013.
11. Vassar MJ, Perry CA, Gannaway WL, et al: 7.5% sodium chloride/dextran for resuscitation of trauma patients undergoing helicopter transport. Arch Surg 1991;126:1065-1072.
12. Boyd M, Vanek VW, Bourguet CC: Emergency room resuscitative thoracotomy: When is it indicated? J Trauma 1992;33:714-721.
13. Fleming A, Bishop M, Shoemaker W: Prospective trial of supranormal values as goals of resuscitation in severe trauma. Arch Surg 1992;127:1175-1181.
14. Shoemaker WC, Appel PL, Kram HB: Prospective trial of supranormal values of survivors as therapeutic goals in high-risk surgical patients. Chest 1988;94:1176-1186.
15. Barone JE, Lowenfels AB: Maximization of oxygen delivery: A plea for moderation. J Trauma 1992:651-653.
16. Gutierrez G: Cellular energy metabolism during hypoxia. Crit Care Med 1991;19:619-626.
17. Peitzman AB, Udekwu AO, Ochoa J: Bacterial translocation in trauma patients. J Trauma 1991;31:1083-1087.
18. Moore FA, Moore EE, Poggetti R: Gut bacterial translocation via the portal vein: A clinical perspective with major torso trauma. J Trauma 1991;31:628-629.
19. Moore FA, Moore EE, Jones TN, et al: TEN versus TPN following major abdominal trauma reduced septic morbidity. J Trauma 1989;29:916-923.

20. Daly JM, Lieberman MD, Goldfine J, et al: Enteral nutrition with supplemental arginine, RNA, and omega-3 fatty acids in patients after operation: Immunologic, metabolic, and clinical outcome. Surg 1992;112:56-67.
21. Fry DE: Multiple system organ failure. Surg Clin North Am 1983;66:107-122.
22. Baue AE, Faist E: What's new in multiple system organ failure. Adv Trauma 1992;7:1-21.

TRANSFUSION GUIDELINES FOR ELECTIVE SURGERY: THE TRANSFUSION TRIGGER

Richard K. Spence, M.D.

University of Medicine and Dentistry of New Jersey
Robert Wood Johnson Medical School at Camden
Cooper Hospital/University Medical Center
Camden, New Jersey

The National Institutes of Health consensus conference, convened in 1988 to address the topic of perioperative red cell transfusion, focused primarily on the risks of transfusion and the need to modify our transfusion practices.[1] It also produced recommendations for a new transfusion trigger that represented an update over the tradtional 10/30 rule that had existed for years. The target, or trigger, hemoglobin was lowered to 8 g/dL and guidelines for transfusion were given that directed attention toward assessment of clinical need and symptoms rather than numbers alone. Since then, much has appeared in the literature that has attempted to further define the transfusion trigger. Investigators have focused on either defining an optimal or minimally acceptable hemoglobin level, deriving a trigger from oxygen transport or metabolic variables, or describing the effect of transfusion in specific clinical settings. In the following section, I have reviewed and summarized relevant information in an attempt to provide the practicing surgeon with both transfusion guidelines and an appreciation of the complexity of the issue. (Table 1)

Two concepts form the basis for the use of hemoglobin as a transfusion trigger, i.e., the optimal hemoglobin/hematocrit and the minimally-acceptable hemoglobin/hematocrit. For many years, they were considered to be one and the same. At the turn of the century, before blood transfusion was possible, surgeons tolerated low hemoglobin levels because there was little one could do to change them. The scientific investigation of blood-oxygen delivery mechanics was in its infancy, transfusion was a very young discipline and little was known about optimal or minimal hemoglobin levels. By the 1930's, Carrel and Lindberg had demonstrated that isolated organs could survive and grow in an extremely anemic environment, defining the minimally-acceptable hemoglobin level for sustained life as approximately 3 g/dL.[2] During the ensuing years, as transfusion became a part of everyday

Critical Issues in Surgery, Edited by A. C. Cernaianu et al.
Plenum Press, New York, 1995

95

Table 1. Approaches to the
Transfusion Trigger

1. Hemoglobin/hematocrit level
2. Oxygen delivery/consumption
3. Oxygen extraction ratio
4. Tissue oxygen debt
5. Lactate levels
6. PvO_2/SvO_2
7. Patient history
8. Cardiac status

practice, the optimal hemoglobin level was defined clinically. In 1941, less than 10 years after the first blood bank opened, Adams and Lundy recommended that all patients with preoperative hemoglobin levels below 10 g/dL be transfused prior to surgery, basing this decision on his clinical experience and understanding of oxygen transport dynamics.[3] A few years later, Clark et al [4] provided some clinical support for the 10 g/dL level when he proposed that patients with the anemia of "chronic shock" would benefit from preoperative transfusion. The 10 g/dL hemoglobin level, or the "10/30" rule for transfusion soon became a doctrine that persisted for many years.

Subsequent studies of the role of hematocrit, cardiac function and oxygen transport have supported 10 g/dL hemoglobin as an optimal level as well. In vitro rheologic studies of diluted blood pumped through glass tubes at constant pressure showed that oxygen delivery (DO_2) peaks at hematocrit levels of 30 percent, then declines with progressive hemodilution.[5] Oxygen transport and survival are maximized at hematocrit levels of 30 to 40 percent in the experimental animal.[6,7] Czer and Shoemaker determined that an optimal hematocrit of 33 percent was desirable in critically ill patients, but emphasized the importance of maintaining adequate volume status over transfusion.[8] Their patients had had acute blood loss from trauma or had undergone emergency surgery. Hemoglobin levels were confounded in their analysis by both the nature of the critical illness and volume replacement. Even so, patients with normal compensatory mechanisms tolerated hematocrit levels as low as 18 percent. These investigators subsequently demonstrated maintainence of both cardiac output and oxygen consumption (VO_2) in dogs with hematocrit levels as low as 10 percent as long as volume remained normal.[9]

Several studies designed to establish an optimal hemoglobin noted that lower levels were tolerated by most patients. Clinical studies give us further information regarding the minimally-acceptable hemoglobin level in the form of mortality and morbidity data in anemic surgical patients. Lunn and Elwood described the mortality rate in 1584 surgical patients who received anesthesia.[10] As the hemoglobin level decreased, the mortality increased. However, this study did not assess or control for other factors that have an effect on survival, i.e., concurrent medical problems or type of surgical procedure. Furthermore, mortality rates were not described for different hemoglobin levels below 10 g/dL, making it impossible to assess the effect of severe anemia on the risk of death. In Rawstron's comparison of 145 patients with preoperative hemoglobin levels less than 10 g/dL to a group of 412 surgical patients with hemoglobin levels 10 g/dL or greater, the number of postoperative complications was similar.[11] However, both groups received perioprative transfusion, which may have obscured a difference in operative risk. Outcomes were not stratified for hemoglobin levels below 10 g/dL. Alexiu compared the postoperative mortality and morbidity in patients with gastrointestinal bleeding.[12] Sixty-nine transfused patients were compared to 72 who were resuscitated with large volumes of dextrose and normal saline. In patients not given blood, the mean preoperative hematocrit was 29 percent (range 16 to 42 percent) , dropping by the second postoperative day to a mean of 23.3 percent (range 10 to 37 percent). There was no mortality and the complication rate was lower than in the transfused group. However, the number of patients with hemoglobin levels below 10 g/dL was not stated and the presence of potentially confounding medical problems was not included.

We have reported two studies of anemia and the risk of postoperative morbidity and mortality in Jehovah's Witnesses.[13,14] In the first study of 125 patients undergoing either emergency or elective surgery, the mean preoperative hemoglobin level in those who died was 7.6 g/dL and was significantly lower than that in the survivors (11.8 g/dL, p<0.002). The percentage of patients who died with preoperative hemoglobin levels between zero to 6 g/dL was 61.5 percent, between 6.1 to 8 g/dL was 33.3 percent, between 8.1 to 10 g/dL was 0 percent and greater than 10 g/dL was 7.1 percent. None of the patients with preoperative hemoglobin levels greater than 8 g/dL and operative blood loss less than 500 mL died (upper 95 percent confidence interval, 5 percent). However, the study was too small to precisely describe the risk of death in patients with hemoglobin levels between 6 g/dL and 10 g/dL. Our subsequent analysis of 113 elective operations in 107 Jehovah's witness patients showed that mortality was zero with hemoglobin levels as low as 6 g/dL as long as blood loss was kept below 500 mL.

Because humans tolerate anemia surprisingly well, symptoms and signs caused by decreased red cell mass have limited uselfulness as transfusion triggers.[15] Symptoms of exertional dyspnea do not appear in the otherwise healthy individual until hemoglobin concentration reaches 7 g/dL. Even at this and lower levels, symptoms and signs are variable. Carmel and Shulman reported on the correlation between symptoms and the need for transfusion in 122 medical patients with pernicious anemia.[16] Sixty-two patients with a mean hemoglobin level of 5.5 g/dL were transfused, but only 34 (55 percent) had symptoms of chest pain, dyspnea at rest, syncope or lethargy suggesting an urgent need for additional blood. Muller and colleagues evaluated the use of a 6 g/dL hemoglobin or 20 percent hematocrit transfusion trigger in 171 patients (100 children, 71 adults).[17] Adults were more likely to demonstrate hemodynamic symptoms at this level of anemia than children, whose predominant symptoms were dyspnea and impaired consciousness. In spite of the severity of the anemia, only 54 percent of all patients were tachycardic, 32 percent were hypotensive, 27 percent had dyspnea and 35 percent had impaired levels of consciousness.

The above studies show that a hemoglobin value significantly lower than an optimal level of 10 g/dL is tolerated by many patients. This does not necessarily mean that a tolerable hemoglobin level should automatically be considered an acceptable level for use as a transfusion trigger in all patients. Conversely, it is unnecessary and potentially risky to transfuse all patients to an optimal hemoglobin of 10 g/dL. The main problem with a hemoglobin-based trigger is its lack of generalizability. Some patients can tolerate very low perioperative hemoglobin levels; others will require supranormal values to survive, depending upon diagnosis and clinical condition.

The use of a minimally-acceptable hemoglobin level as a transfusion trigger assumes that all patients are able to mobilize compensatory mechanisms equally and adequately. This may not be the case, especially in those patients with underlying coronary artery disease. The heart is more dependent on delivery for its oxygen supply than other organs, extracting approximately one-half its delivery. When hemoglobin falls, an increase in cardiac output requires a concomitant increase in coronary artery blood flow. In the presence of critical coronary artery stenoses, the heart may be unable to respond sufficiently to meet its oxygen demands, leading to ischemia.[19] Animal studies of normovolemic hemodilution have shown that the lower limit of cardiac tolerance for anemia lies around 3 to 5 g/dL.[18-20] Under these conditions, coronary blood flow is shifted from the endocardium to the epicardium, thereby placing subendocardial tissue at an increased risk of ischemia. The addition of an experimental coronary stenosis to this model results in depressed cardiac function at hemoglobin levels of 7 to 10 g/dL.

The minimally-acceptable hemoglobin may be that beyond which coronary artery blood flow can not increase enough to meet myocardial oxygen demands, but this level has yet to be defined in useful clinical terms.[6] Robertie and Gravlie recommend accepting a transfusion trigger of 6 g/dL in well-compensated patients with no cardiac disease and no postoperative complications.[6] A higher trigger, i.e., 8 g/dL, should be used in patients with stable cardiac disease and when blood loss of approximately 300 cc is expected. Older patients and those with postoperative complications who can not increase cardiac output to compensate for hemodilution should be transfused when hemoglobin reaches 10 g/dL. There have been few clinical studies of the effect of co-existing medical conditions on the ability of the heart to compensate for moderate or severe anemia. In our study of mortality and hemoglobin level in Jehovah's Witnesses, preoperative cardiac disease as defined by the Multifactorial Cardiac Risk Index appeared to worsen outcome.[14] In a smaller study of 47 patients with more severe anemia (mean Hb 4.6±.2 g/dL), a history of cardiac, pulmonary or renal disease had no association with adverse outcome.[21] Two recent reports of an increased incidence of electrocardiographic evidence of myocardial ischemia in postoperative vascular patients with hematocrits below 29 percent are worrisome, although neither accounted for the presence or severity of underlying heart disease.[22,23] All of these studies are limited by small numbers.

Dissatisfaction with the use of either an optimal or a minimally-acceptable hemoglobin-derived transfusion trigger have lead to a search for a physiologically-defined trigger based on oxygen-derived variables. In most clinical settings, oxygen consumption is relatively independent of hemoglobin level across a wide range of oxygen delivery values because of compensations made in oxygen extraction. As DO_2 decreases through a loss of hemoglobin, oxygen extraction should increase from a baseline of 15-25 percent to maintain a constant consumption. Any increase in circulating volume that improves cardiac output will also mathematically improve oxygen delivery regardless of hemoglobin level. (Table 2) However, an

Table 2. Hemoglobin and Oxygen Interactions

Cardiac Output (CO) = Stroke Volume (SV) x Heart Rate (HR)
Oxygen Content (CaO_2) = (1.39 X SO_2 X Hb + 0.003 X PO_2) X 10mL O_2/L

where:

SO_2 = oxygen saturation and   Hb = Hemoglobin concentration in g/dL
Oxygen Delivery (DO_2) = CO X CaO_2 mL O_2/min
Oxygen Consumption (VO_2) = CO X (CaO_2-CvO_2) mL O_2/min

improvement in DO_2 does not necessarily lead to an increase in oxygen consumption.

Wilkerson et al have shown in the exchange-transfused baboon that VO_2 is maintained down to an hematocrit of 4 percent if left atrial pressure is held constant.[24] These animals survived by increasing their oxygen extraction ratio significantly. The investigators detected a conversion to anaerobic metabolism at a 10 percent hematocrit level which correlated with an O_2ER of 50 percent, suggesting these two numbers might be useful as transfusion guidelines. We found similar results in a study of 12 nontransfused, postsurgical patients with a mean hematocrit of 7.5 percent. O_2ER was greater than 50 percent in the first 48 hours in nonsurvivors, a level that was significantly higher than in those who lived. Hematocrit was also lower—6.0 vs 9.6 percent—in nonsurvivors.

From the formulae for oxygen content and oxygen consumption (Table 2), it would seem that as hemoglobin levels increase, both DO_2 and VO_2 should increase. Although increasing hemoglobin level does lead to higher DO_2 because of added blood volume, this does not always guarantee a rise in VO_2. Table 3 summarizes the major studies that have been conducted to evaluate the effect of transfusion on oxygen transport. These patients run the gamut from postoperative surgical patients[25-34] to those with recent hemorrhage,[29] burns,[30] cardiogenic shock[32] and sepsis.[25-28,33] Pretransfusion oxygen extraction ratio ranges between 24 to 48 percent, with the highest values seen in patients with cardiogenic shock. The effect of transfusion to a hemoglobin level of 10 g/dL on oxygen extraction ratio was minimal in most patients. Moreover, although transfusion increased oxygen delivery in all patients, only half the groups showed an increase in oxygen comsumption, with the other half showing no change. These differences may be caused by the linear relationship between oxygen delivery and consumption that exists in patients with septic and cardiogenic shock.[28] Regardless of the cause, they point out the lack of precision in the use of a predefined oxygen extraction ratio or similar variable as a transfusion trigger.

Sepsis and anemia is a particularly lethal combination as suggested by our study which included 12 septic patients with hemoglobin levels below 5 g/dL, all of whom died.[21] This corroborates Shoemaker's finding that survival is decreased in sepsis when VO_2 is compromised, in part because of increased tissue oxygen debt and a resetting of DO_2/VO_2 interactions.[28] Although his work suggests that transfusing to supranormal hematocrits may be beneficial, transfusion has not always turned the tide in sepsis. (Table 3) It may be that giving additional blood to the compromised, septic

Table 3. Effect of Transfusion in Critically Ill Patients

Author	Number	Diagnosis	VO$_2$ Pre	VO$_2$ Post	DO$_2$ Pre	DO$_2$ Post	O$_2$ Pre	O$_2$ Post	H/H Pre	H/H Post
McCormick (29)	14	Blood loss	494	599	143	140	30	24	27.9	36.7
Dietrich (31)	36	19 sepsis; 14 cardio shock; 3 other	410	525	119	118	30.8	23.7	8.3	10.5
Babineau (25)	30	Postop	401	433	117	115	31	28	9.4	10.4
Marino (26)	20	Postop	281	329	109	110	39	33	7.1	8.6
Robbins (27)	58	ICU	331	430	115	141	36	35	8.75	—
Steffes (32)	21	Sepsis	532	634	145	160	27	25	9.3	10.7
Gore (30)	5	Burn	882	1060	199	206	24	20	7.5	10.5
Shoemaker (28)	69	Sepsis	467	529	132	154	30	29	27.6	32.0
Shoemaker (128)	132	ICU	470	562	132	156	28	28	—	—

DO$_2$ = oxygen delivery; VO$_2$ = oxygen consumption; O$_2$ ER = oxygen extraction ratio; H/H = hemoglobin/hematocrit; pre = pretransfusion; post = post transfusion

patient to improve oxygen delivery cannot compensate alone for the increased tissue oxygen debt.

Other approaches to defining the transfusion trigger in metabolic terms have had limited success. Bihari et al[34] have shown that patients with ARDS may have a hidden oxygen debt unrelated to hemoglobin level. They used prostacyclin administration to define DO$_2$/VO$_2$ relationships in hopes of identifying those patients who would benefit from additional oxygen, but this test has not gained widespread use. Lactate levels have not been helpful in defining transfusion need. Astiz et al[35] found no correlation between lactate and oxygen delivery in 100 patients with either an acute myocardial infarction or sepsis. The role of PvO$_2$ and SvO$_2$ as triggers have yet to be defined.

From this brief investigation of the transfusion trigger, we can conclude that there is inadequate data to recommend a specific transfusion trigger based on either hemoglobin level or oxygen transport variables. Neither optimal nor minimally-acceptable hemoglobin levels are useful as a trigger because of both under and overestimation of transfusion need. Clinical symptoms of cardiac compromise or decreased DO$_2$ do not correlate well with hemoglobin levels. Oxygen transport derived transfusion triggers such as extraction ratio are both organ and setting specific, with no consistent correlation to either hemoglobin level or red cell transfusion, and significant changes appear late in the game. In the critically ill ICU patient where invasive monitoring is justifiable, measurements of oxygen transport variables may be useful.

In summary, the decision to transfuse should be related to the specific patients needs and condition. The presence of cardiac, pulmonary and other atherosclerotic disease processes should be assessed and quantified when possible. Patients with coronary artery disease and pulmonary hypoxia will most likely require higher perioperative hemoglobin levels than those with normal hearts and lungs to avoid ischemia and undue cardiac stress.

REFERENCES

1. Perioperative red cell transfusion. NIH consensus development conference statement: 1988;7(4):1-17.
2. Diamond LK: A history of blood transfusion in blood, pure and eloquent. Wintrobe MM (ed), McGraw-Hill, New York, NY. 1908:659-683.
3. Adams RC, Lundy JS: Anesthesia in cases of poor surgical risk. Some suggestions for decreasing the risk. Surg Gyn Obst 1942;74:1011-1019.
4. Clark JH, Nelson W, Lyons C, et al: Chronic shock: the problem of reduced blood volume in the chronically ill patient. Ann Surg 1947;125:618.
5. Stehling L, Zauder HL: Acute normovolemic hemodilution. Transfusion 1991;31(9):857-868.
6. Robertie PG, Gravlee GP: Safe limits of hemodiltuion and recommendations for erythrocyte transfusion. Int Anesthesiol Clin 1990:28(4):197-204.
7. Chapler CK, Cain SM: The physiologic reserve in oxygen carrying capacity: studies in experimental hemodilution. Can J Physiol Pharmacol 1986;64:7-12.
8. Czer LSC, Shoemaker WC: Optimal hematocrit value in critically ill postoperative patients. Surg Gynec Obstet 1978;147:363-8.
9. Schwarz S, Frantz RA, Shoemaker WC: Sequential hemodynamic and oxygen transport responses in hypovolemia, anemia, and hypoxia. Am J Physiol 1981;241:(Heart Circ Physiol 10):HH64-HH72.
10. Lunn JN, Elwood PC: Anemia and surgery. Br Med J 1970;3:71-3.
11. Rawstron ER: Anemia and surgery: a retrospective clinical study. Aust NZ J Surg 1970;39:425-32.
12. Alexiu O, Mircea N, Balaban M, et al: Gastrointestinal hemorrhage from peptic ulcer: an evaluation of bloodless transfusion and early surgery. Anaesthesia 1975;30:609-15.
13. Spence RK, Carson JA, Poses R, et al: Elective surgery without transfusion: influence of preoperative hemoglobin level and blood loss on mortality. Am J Surg 1990;59:320-4.
14. Carson JL, Spence RK, Poses RM, et al: Severity of anemia and operative mortality and morbidity. Lancet 1988;2:727-9.
15. Linman JW: Physiologic and pathophysiologic effects of anemia. N Eng J Med 1968;279:812-818.
16. Carmel R, Shulman IA: Blood transfusion in medically treatable chronic anemia: pernicious anemia as a model for transfusion overuse. Arch Pathol Lab Md 1989;113:995-997.
17. Muller G, N'tita I, Nyst M, et al: Application of blood transfusion guidelines in a major hospital of Kinshasa, Zaire. [letter]AIDS 1992;6(4):431-432.
18. Geha AS, Baue AE: Grade coronary stenosis and coronary flow during acute normovolemic anemia. World J Surg 1978;2:645-51.
19. Buckberg G, Brazier J: Coronary blood flow and cardiac function during hemodilution. Bibl Haematol 1974;41:173-89.
20. Wilkerson DK, Rosen AL, Sehgal LR, et al: Limits of cardiac compensation in anemic baboons. Surgery 1988:103:665-70.
21. Spence RK, Costabile JP, Young GS, et al: Is hemoglobin level alone a reliable predictor of outcome in the severely anemic patient? Amer Surg 1992;58(2):92-95.
22. Nelson AH, Fleisher LA, Rosenbaum SH: The relationship between postoperative anemia and cardiac morbidity in high risk vascular patients in the ICU.[abstract] Crit Care Med 1992;20(4)Suppl.:S71.

23. Christopherson R, Frank S, Norris E et al: Low postoperative hematocrit is associated with cardiac ischemia in high-risk patients.[abstract] Anesthesiology 1991;75(3A):A100.

24. Wilkerson DK, Rosen AL, Gould SA, et al: Oxygen extraction ratio: a valid indicator of myocardial metabolism in anemia. J Surg Res 1987;42:629-34.

25. Babineau TJ, Dzik WH, Borlase BC, et al: Reevaluation of current transfusion practices in surgical intensive care units. Am J Surg 1992;164:22-25.

26. Marino PL, Krasner J: An interpretive computer program for analyzing hemodynamic problems in the ICU. Crit Care Med 198;12:601-4.

27. Robbins J, Keating K, Orlando R, III, et al: Effects of blood transfusion on oxygen consumption and oxygen delivery in critically ill surgical patients.[abstract] Crit Care Med 1992;20(4)Suppl:S113.

28. Shoemaker WC, Appel PL, Kram HB: Tissue oxygen debt as determinant of lethal and non-lethal postoperative organ failure. Crit Care 1988;Med 16:1117-20.

29. McCormick M, Feustel PJ, Newell JC, et al: Effect of cardiac index and hematocrit changes in oxygen consumption in resuscitated patients. J Surg Res 1988;44:499-505.

30. Gore DC, DeMaria EJ, Reines HD: Elevations in red blood cell mass reduce cardiac index without altering the oxygen consumption in severely burnes patients. Surg Forum 1991:721-3.

31. Dietrich KA, Conrad SA, Cullen AH, et al: Cardiovascular and metabolic response to red blood cell transfusion in critically ill volume-resuscitated nonsurgical patients. Crit Care Med 1990;18:940-44.

32. Steffes CP, Bender JS, Levison MA: Blood transfusion and oxygen consumption in surgical sepsis. Crit Care Med 1991;19:512.

33. Edwards JD: Oxygen transport in cardiogenic and septic shock. Crit Care Med 1991;19:658-663

34. Bihari DJ, Tinker J: The therapeutic value of prostaglandins in multiple organ failure associated with sepsis. Intensive Care Med 1988;15(1):2-7.

35. Astiz ME, Rackow EC, Falk JL, et al: Oxygen delivery and consumption in patients with hyperdynamic septic shock. Crit Care Med 1987;15(1):26-8.

PHYSIOLOGIC PREDICTORS OF TRANSFUSION NEED IN THE INTENSIVE CARE UNIT

Loren D. Nelson, M.D.

Vanderbilt University Medical Center
Nashville, Tennessee

Transfusion of blood products plays a major role in optimizing oxygen delivery to tissues. In the 1990s, we have gained a better understanding of the risks and benefits of blood component therapy in critically ill patients. While we are better able to reduce the transmission of viral disease through donor screening and blood testing, we have learned that blood transfusion has significant effects on immune function and may increase risks of tumor recurrence and perioperative bacterial infections.

The question that remains in the care of every critically ill surgical patient is *when do we initiatiate transfusion? What factors should be considered when transfusing red blood cells? What are the physiologic predictors that patients will require blood? When can other solutions be used to replace volume losses? If blood is needed, should it be given early or later?* This chapter will review the physiology of perioperative fluid replacement based on oxygen transport principles which help the clinician predict the need for transfusion of red blood cells.

PERIOPERATIVE FLUID REPLACEMENT

Two basic "rules" govern fluid management in virtually all patients. The first and most important rule is: "replace to the intravascular space what is lost from the intravascular space". In a bleeding patient who is loosing red cells and plasma, appropriate volume replacement must include red cells and plasma. In a patient who is losing fluid into the interstitial space, the resuscitation fluid management must include crystalloid solutions which approximate the electrolyte composition of interstitial fluid.

A second general rule that can be applied to most patients in the perioperative period is to supply replacement fluids with the assumption that homeostasis is more easily restored in an "economy of abundance". In the vast majority of surgical patients over-replacement of estimated fluid losses is well

Critical Issues in Surgery, Edited by A. C. Cernaianu et al.
Plenum Press, New York, 1995

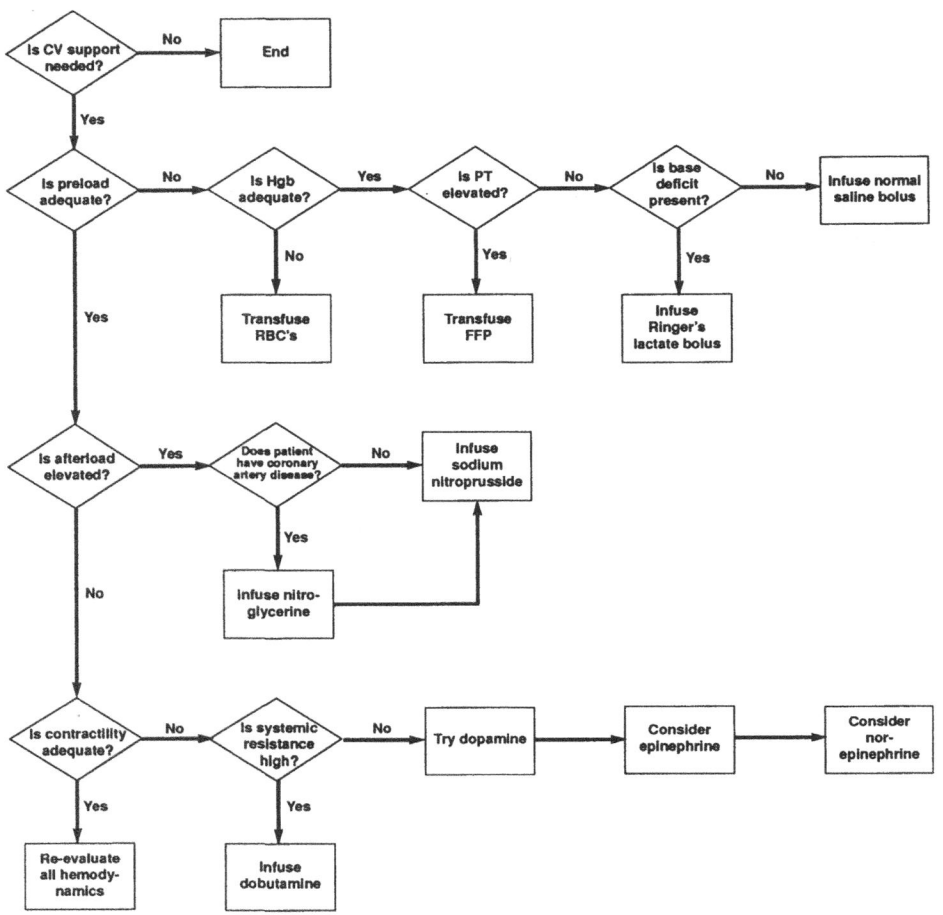

Figure 1. An algorithm for the support of oxygen transport and stroke volume in critically ill patients with a pulmonary artery catheter in place. If cardiovascular (CV) support is needed as determined by oxygen transport variables, preload is augmented, afterload reduced, and contractility enhanced. Preload augmentation is part of the postoperative fluid management in many critically ill surgical patients. Hb = hemoglobin concentration, PT = prothrombin time, RBCs = red blood cells, FFP = fresh frozen plasma.

handled and will result in a brisk diuresis as the patient begins to mobilize fluid. Under-resuscitation with fluid may result in prolongation of a hypoperfused state leading either to shock, worsening organ system dysfunction or failure, or a need for even greater volumes of fluid at a later period of time. Early fluid resuscitation may minimize the sequelae of prolonged hypovolemia and actually decrease the total volume of fluid required by the patient. The *economy of abundance* should not imply that patients should be fluid overloaded. Rather, fluid resuscitation of patients should be tailored to their precise needs with the understanding that under-resuscitation is probably more detrimental in the long term than is over-resuscitation.

The next consideration in the selection of perioperative fluid replacement is the relative priority of different types of fluid (Figure 1). Clearly, the bleeding patient needs blood more than crystalloid. A patient with a significant coagulopathy may need fresh frozen plasma more than albumin and the patient with thrombocytopenia may need platelets more than plasma.

RED BLOOD CELLS

Restoration of a red cell mass is of vital importance in a patient who has had significant hemorrhage. The transfusion of red blood cells not only has the effect of restoring intravascular volume and peripheral perfusion, but also re-establishes oxygen carrying capacity thus improving oxygen delivery more than any other fluid.[19] The transfusion of red cells has additional benefits in that it provides a significant intravascular oncotic load that helps to minimize the flux of fluid from the intravascular space to the interstitium. Red cells have an advantage over other oncotic agents in that the favorable oncotic effect is maintained even in the presence of an extremely low reflection coefficient which allows albumin and other large molecules to leak into the interstitium.

The transfusion of red cells is associated with two clearly delineated risks to the patient. The first risk is that of an immunologically mediated reaction to the red cells, plasma proteins, or potential allergens present in the blood. Modern blood banking techniques have reduced the incidence of major transfusion reactions to well within a clinically acceptable range. Major hemolytic reactions to transfused blood are almost unheard of today and are virtually always related to personnel and clerical errors.[62] Minor allergen related reactions still occur and are usually manifested by fever and/or a rash beginning shortly after the administration of the blood. Very rarely the allergic reaction may precipitate bronchospasm or even laryngospasm which requires aggressive medical treatment. Much more commonly, however, the reaction is terminated by discontinuance of the blood product administration and occasionally the administration of an antihistamine with or without an antipyretic.

The other major concern regarding the transfusion of blood and blood products is the spread of transfusion associated diseases.[1,31,58] The major risks are hepatitis B, hepatitis C, and the human immune deficiency virus (HIV). In the early 1990's the estimated risk of disease transmission from transfused blood is less than 0.1 percent per unit of blood products transfused.

While programs using the directed donation of blood have not apparently reduced the incidence of blood related infection problems significantly, autotransfusion and the preoperative banking of autologus blood has eliminated this risk in certain patients undergoing elective surgical procedures commonly associated with transfusion.[38]

Another concern that has been raised in the late 1980's and early 1990's has been the potential immunosuppression occurring in patients who are transfused with significant amounts of blood. Data regarding the immunosuppressive effects of transfusion are extremely difficult to interpret and are often conflicting.[2,3,12,18,25,32,57,73] It appears that patients who receive significant amounts of blood exhibit a reduced immune response as manifest by increased tolerance to transplantation of solid organs.[66] There is also concern that patients receiving transfusion of significant volumes of blood may be immunosuppressed and be at increased risk for recurrence of certain tumors, most notably those in the head and neck region and in the colon.[94] What is not entirely clear from the literature at this time is whether or not tumor recurrence is related to a larger initial tumor load thus necessitating a greater magnitude of surgery and increased risk of bleeding and thus transfusion. Also it is not entirely clear at this time whether it is transfusion or shock which predisposes the patients to a depressed immunologic response.[18]

It is probably fair to summarize that patients manifesting significant signs of impaired oxygen transport related to decreased in intravascular volume compounded by decreased oxygen carrying capacity should receive red blood cells to improve total body oxygen delivery.[27,68,91,93]

FRESH FROZEN PLASMA

Indications for fresh frozen plasma in postoperative patients are relatively clear.[37] Patients who have a significant coagulopathy as manifest by prolonged prothrombin time, who are bleeding, or who are at significant risk for bleeding have a medical indication for fresh frozen plasma. Fresh frozen plasma should not be used for restoration of intravascular volume in patients with no evidence of coagulopathy or active bleeding. Fresh frozen plasma may be used to reverse the effects of Coumadin and related anticoagulants in patients who are bleeding or require emergency surgical procedures. These anticoagulants may also be reversed by parenteral administration of vitamin K when intravascular volume, active bleeding, and the need for re-anticoagulation are not significant clinical concerns.

Administration of fresh frozen plasma to patients at risk for large volume blood losses who are being transfused with packed red cells (rather than whole blood) may be prudent.[17,35,37,38,53] However, dilutional coagulopathies from large volume transfusions rarely result from the loss of clotting factors in patients without underlying coagulopathy or significant liver disease. Bleeding related to massive transfusion is much more commonly associated with a dilutional thrombocytopenia or hypothermia.[71,85]

OTHER BLOOD PRODUCTS

Other blood products occasionally need to be transfused in the patient receiving large volumes of red cells for persistent bleeding or hemorrhagic shock. The most common blood product is platelets for persistent bleeding in patients with dilutional thrombocytopenia, acquired platelet dysfunction, or persistent bleeding while being actively transfused large volumes of red cells.[15,17] The indications for platelet transfusion generally are not based solely upon the total platelet count.[71] However, some guidelines are available based on the platelet count in patients who are not bleeding. Spontaneous onset of bleeding is extremely uncommon in adult patients with functional platelets whose counts exceed 20,000/mm^3. Patients at high risk for bleeding complications probably should be transfused platelets to keep the total platelet count greater than 50,000/mm^3. Patients with active bleeding who are being transfused probably should receive platelets to maintain the total platelet count greater than 100,000/mm^{3}.[95]

When a clinical indication for platelet transfusion has been identified, the dose of platelets should be tailored to the patient's size. Generally one unit of platelets is transfused for every 10 kg of patient body weight. This dose of platelets should raise the total platelet count by approximately 50,000/mm^{3}. An increase of less than 50,000 with this dose of platelets implies on going platelet sequestration or consumption. This dose of platelets may be repeated as necessary depending on the patient's bleeding status and platelet count.

Assessment of platelet dysfunction in surgical patients is often difficult and precise tests for platelet function are often available only in specialized laboratories. When there is no evidence of significant coagulopathy (i.e., prothrombin time and partial thromboplastin times are normal) and the total platelet count is greater than 100,000/mm^{3}, the bleeding time may be a useful test to assess the adequacy of platelet function. In the absence of other coagulopathies and a normal platelet count, a bleeding time in excess of nine minutes may be suggestive of platelet dysfunction. A bleeding time of less than six minutes rules out significant coagulopathy or platelet dysfunction in most patients.

Cryoprecipitate is occasionally indicated in the patient who is bleeding or is at great risk for bleeding from factor VIII deficiency or from a severe consumption coagulopathy and decreased fibrinogen. While concentrated factor VIII is probably the primary therapy for a hemophiliac patient who is bleeding or at great risk for bleeding, cryoprecipitate may also serve as a source of this factor. Cryoprecipitate is also the most concentrated source for fibrinogen for patients who have a consumptive coagulopathy, have not responded to fresh frozen plasma, and are showing hypofibrinogenemia. The dose of cryoprecipitate which is often used to replace fibrinogen is ten units.

ALBUMIN AND OTHER COLLOIDS

The administration of albumin and other colloid solutions as part of the postoperative fluid management of patients remains controversial.[8,20,70] The two points upon which nearly all agree are: 1) colloids are significantly more expensive than crystalloids and, 2) colloids are more efficient in acutely increasing intravascular volume.[70,82]

Numerous clinical and basic studies have demonstrated that colloid administration is approximately three fold more efficient in the restoration of intravascular volume than crystalloid administration. This means that approximately one-third of the resuscitation volume can be administered using colloid rather than crystalloid. The increased efficiency of colloid in raising intravascular volume carries the risk of intravascular fluid overload and hydrostatic pulmonary edema.[50,56,75,90] The implication of using colloid in the resuscitation of hypovolemic shock following surgery is that very careful clinical monitoring must be performed to prevent intravascular fluid overload. A number of prospective randomized clinical trials have compared a pure crystalloid resuscitation with a combined crystalloid and colloid resuscitation in both surgical and nonsurgical patients. There are reported

advantages and disadvantages of each resuscitation regimen that differ
between the trials. Some of these differences are due to patient selection
and other differences to the physiologic end-points selected for resuscitation
and perhaps the type of fluid administered.[89] One of the more interesting
overviews aimed at settling the controversy regarding the use of colloid
solutions in the fluid management of critically ill patients was performed
by Velanovich.[88] This metanalysis of the prospective randomized trials
looked at specific resuscitation end-points and outcome using crystalloid
or a crystalloid/colloid combination in the resuscitation of patients. While
there were many conclusions drawn from this metanalysis, the most
striking feature seemed to be an outcome (i.e., mortality) advantage of pure
crystalloid solutions in surgical patients and an outcome advantage of
mixed crystalloid/colloid resuscitations in medical patients. The differences
were statistically significant although the clinical implications of the
metanalysis are not entirely clear.

It is easy to understand why there may be an outcome advantage
of colloid over crystalloid since it more efficiently expands the intravascular
volume.[51] Two questions, however, continue to arise when colloid resuscitations are considered. The first question is regarding whether or not
colloids are worth the great increase in patient cost incurred by their use.
Colloids are approximately 15 - 60 fold more expensive than crystalloid
on a volume basis. When the efficiency factor is included, colloids will
still cost 5 - 15 times as much as crystalloid used to similar resuscitation
end-points.

The other major problem plaguing the advocates of a colloid resuscitation is evidence that albumin may have detrimental effects on end-organ function. Several studies have demonstrated an impairment in
coagulation following colloid administration.[14,42,48,49] Additional studies
have shown rather unequivocal evidence that albumin administration
impairs renal function[52,81] and the ability of the kidney to excrete sodium.
Other studies have demonstrated a possible adverse effect on myocardial
contractility[21,46] and vasodilatation[9] using commercially prepared albumin
solutions. Finally, a number of studies suggest that pulmonary function
is more severely compromised using an albumin resuscitation versus a
pure crystalloid resuscitation.[29,29,40,50,56,90,92] The two hypothesis regarding
impairment of pulmonary function include a propensity to develop hydrostatic pulmonary edema from over-resuscitation when albumin solutions
are used. The second pulmonary problem encountered with the use of
colloids in patients with permeability defects in the microvasculature of
the lung is the potential for increased colloid oncotic pressures in the
lung interstitium as colloid leaks through the endothelium.[60] The presence
of colloid in the pulmonary interstitium or alveoli theoretically may pull
more fluid into these spaces and may prolong the need for mechanical
ventilation.

When patients have high albumin and protein losses due to reaccu-
mulation of ascites, pleural effusions, or extrinsic losses from burns and
other soft tissue injuries, it would seem appropriate to replace these
albumin losses with albumin solutions. It would also seem prudent to
replace albumin in the resuscitation of patients who have marked impairment of hepatic albumin synthesis. However, in the vast majority of post-

operative patients colloid containing solutions have little or no role, are quite costly, and show no benefit in improving patient outcome.

CRYSTALLOID SOLUTIONS

Sodium containing crystalloid solutions are the mainstay of perioperative fluid management. These solutions may be tailored to meet precise electrolyte and volume requirements in a variety of clinical situations and may be used to meet insensible fluid losses, measurable fluid losses and the third space fluid losses acquired by critically ill surgical patients.

The initial studies showing the improved efficacy of crystalloid resuscitation in hypovolemic shock were performed by Shires in the 1960's.[76,78] His carefully controlled animal and clinical studies demonstrated an improvement in outcome when resuscitation was continued to normalize not only the intravascular volume but also the interstitial volume. When animals were resuscitated after a period of hemorrhagic shock with all of their shed blood, the mortality was 80 percent. When animals were resuscitated with all of their shed blood plus a volume of plasma estimated to normalize the intravascular volume, the mortality remained at 70 percent. When the animals were given their shed blood plus a volume of balanced salt solution with the approximate composition of interstitial fluid to a volume which normalized *interstitial* volume the mortality fell dramatically to 30 percent. These results led Shires and others to advocate resuscitation of shock with a combination of the estimated volume of blood which had been lost by the patient plus balance salt solution to normalize hemodynamics.[10,11,30,77,78]

It is clear that resuscitation of hypovolemic shock to restore interstitial volume is of great importance in critically ill postoperative patients. What is beginning to become apparent is that restoration of the interstitial sodium concentration may be of greater importance. Recent studies using hypertonic saline resuscitations have demonstrated that smaller resuscitation volumes may be used to reach similar physiologic end-points.[4,6,16,33] The advantage of hypertonic solutions over isotonic solutions is that in patients who have very large volume requirements, the total amount of fluid of administered may be decreased.[59,61] Generally, when solutions containing approximately twice the sodium concentration of normal saline are used, approximately half of the volume may be used to reach the same physiologic end-point. There seems to be a significant benefit of hypertonic solutions in reducing post-resuscitation edema. Hypertonic solutions have been used in the resuscitation of patients with major burns,[59,61] severe closed head injuries,[28,69,83,84] and hypovolemic shock.[67] Although these solutions are clearly associated with a lower resuscitation volume load, the effect on patient outcome and mortality has yet to be delineated.[86,87]

ASSESSMENT OF VOLUME REQUIREMENTS

Once it has been determined that the patient is having significant volume losses in the postoperative period, the nature of those fluid losses must be determined. As indicated earlier, insensible losses are generally easy to estimate and may be replaced primarily with free water and a very small amount of sodium. Measurable losses can be calculated and, when the electrolyte composition of the fluid loss is in question, it can be measured directly. The most difficult assessment of fluid loss comes in estimating third space fluid losses caused by direct injury, shock, or sepsis.

Three general means have been used to assess the adequacy of circulating volume and adequacy of resuscitation following trauma or major surgical procedures. These three assessments include general end-organ perfusion, hemodynamic monitoring, and oxygen transport monitoring.[23]

GENERAL END-ORGAN PERFUSION

In the vast majority of surgical patients the only assessment of intravascular volume that is necessary is a general assessment of end-organ perfusion. The end-organs commonly reviewed include brain, skin, and kidneys. Assessment of these systems coupled with measurement of vital signs and response to fluid challenges are adequate indicators of circulating volume in more than 90 percent of surgical patients.

When mental status is completely normal, cerebral perfusion is usually well maintained. Unfortunately, in most surgical patients mental status is difficult to assess because of residual effects of anesthetics, narcotics, sedatives, and other drugs. Also, cerebral perfusion is maintained well into the later stages of hypovolemic shock. Most of the body's compensatory mechanisms are aimed at maintaining cerebral perfusion and, therefore, central nervous system status often does not change until shock is in a rather advanced stage.

The assessment of cutaneous perfusion has often been used to assess the adequacy of circulatory volume. A patients whose skin is warm, pink, and shows good capillary refill generally has an adequate circulating volume present. However, states associated with vasoderegulation such as sepsis, spinal cord injury, and regional anesthetics often cause a significant maldistribution of blood flow favoring skin perfusion at the expense of more vital organs. In these patients, warm and pink may actually imply a worsening in their vasoregulatory state. Furthermore, patients with acute and chronic vascular disease may show markedly impaired cutaneous perfusion when central perfusion is, in fact, totally adequate.

Monitoring of urinary output and renal function is probably the most important clinical indicator of the adequacy of circulating volume. Patients who have normal vital signs and adequate urine output are generally well perfused. A number of factors may increase urine output pathologically even in conditions of relative intravascular volume depletion: osmotic diuretics (hyperglycemia and glycosuria, intravenous contrast agents, mannitol, large amounts of sodium associated with a volume resuscitation, alcohol), nonoliguric acute renal insufficiency,[7] loop diuretic agents, vasopressors and inotropes. A careful assessment of the patient may be necessary to determine that what is normally an "adequate" urine output is, in fact, so.

HEMODYNAMIC MEASUREMENTS IN THE ASSESSMENT OF INTRAVASCULAR VOLUME

Traditional vital signs are essential in the assessment of the adequacy of circulating volume. Heart rate, blood pressure, and the response of these variables to a change in body position are part of the routine assessment in nearly all surgical patients. In the absence of significant underlying heart disease and medications which alter normal cardiovascular reflexes, the presence of a normal blood pressure and a slow heart rate generally implies an adequate circulatory volume. In the presence of significant cardiac disease or medications affecting the autonomic nervous system and normal cardiovascular reflexes, the interpretation of pulse and blood pressure in the assessment of circulatory volume must be done with caution.

Tachycardia is a relatively sensitive but extremely non-specific response. Tachycardia usually occurs with intravascular volume depletion and shock but also may be caused by pain, anxiety, agitation, fever, hypoxemia, hypercarbia, acidemia, and a variety of other abnormalities often seen in critically ill postoperative patients. The presence of tachycardia therefore should be a red flag alerting the clinical care team to look further into the cause of the tachycardia.

Blood pressure is of such fundamental importance that many of the body's autonomic responses are geared specifically to its maintenance. Baroreceptors present in the carotid sinus and aortic arch trigger reflexes to induce vasoconstriction, tachycardia, and increases in contractility of the myocardium to maintain blood pressure until volume depletion is so severe that the homeostatic mechanisms fail. Waiting for blood pressure changes to indicate intravascular volume depletion results in significant delays in appropriate treatment and may compromise the patient's outcome.

Because of the problems associated with the assessment of general perfusion status, end-organ function, and traditional vital signs, clinicians have searched for other means to detect hypovolemia at an early point in time. The so called "tilt test" is useful in some patients to demonstrate the inability to fully compensate for a decreased circulating volume. In the absence of medications which impair autonomic nervous system function and hemodynamic response to stress, raising the head of a hypovolemic patient will usually induce tachycardia and perhaps lower blood pressure. Generally, this is an indication of marginal or compromised circulating intravascular volume.

In spite of all of the non-invasive assessment means available to the clinician, a small number of postoperative patients will need invasive hemodynamic monitoring to better assess their intravascular volume status and the adequacy of perfusion.[23,41,54] Complete hemodynamic monitoring may also be necessary to guide fluid administration in complex postoperative patients with multiple organ system dysfunction or failure. In the early 1990s complete hemodynamic monitoring implies placement of a flow-directed pulmonary artery catheter capable of measuring intravascular pressures and cardiac output.[79] One of the most difficult issues associated with pulmonary artery catheterization is determining the adequacy and appropriateness of the measured values in an individual patient. The goal of hemodynamic monitoring is to provide a database which will give the clinician information which can be used to optimize the delivery of oxygen and other substrates to meet the requirements of metabolically active tissues.

Cardiac output is determined by the heart rate and stroke volume which is dependent upon the interaction between preload, afterload, and contractility. There are no normal values for cardiac output and only wide ranges of normal cardiac indices adjusted for the body surface area of the patient. Since blood pressure is relatively constant in most healthy patients, metabolic demands determined by tissue mass necessitate variations in cardiac output according to the patient's size. Since there are no normal values for cardiac output, all of the variables used to assess normal hemodynamics must be based upon cardiac index and, therefore, the size of the patient.

The single most important determinant of stroke volume index is cardiac preload. Preload is defined by the fiber length of the cardiac myofibrils at end-diastole. Since the fiber length is directly related to the end-diastolic volume, this value may be used as an indicator of ventricular preload. For many of the more than 20 years that the flow-directed pulmonary artery catheter has been available, many clinicians have assumed that ventricular compliance is relatively fixed and therefore, end-diastolic pressures, to some degree, reflect preload. Commonly, the pulmonary artery occlusion pressure (PAOP), often erroneously referred to as the pulmonary capillary wedge pressure, has been used as an indication of left ventricular end-diastolic pressure. This assumption is generally valid if the catheter is properly positioned, the measurements are carefully transduced, and there is no significant mitral valve disease. A patient who has an inadequate cardiac index and a low PAOP is, therefore, generally believed to be intravascularly volume depleted. A volume challenge may be given with the intent of improving cardiac index by raising the ventricular end-diastolic volume (Figure 1). This assumption is generally valid as long as pulmonary artery occlusion pressure is low.

Elevations in PAOP may be caused by an absolute increase in circulating volume, a decrease in left ventricular function, or an increase in intrathoracic pressure caused by positive pressure mechanical ventilation. Therefore, a low PAOP in a patient with inadequate cardiac output, can generally be assumed to be an indicator of volume depletion and a volume challenge may be safely applied. Patients with high PAOP are much more difficult problems since a high PAOP is not necessarily associated with an increased or even adequate ventricular end-diastolic volume. A high PAOP is often associated with intravascular volume overload if intrapleural pressures and left ventricular function are normal.

Because of the difficulty in interpreting pressure measurements as an indicator of preload, new technology has become available to assess ventricular end-diastolic volume using a thermodilution technique.[72] This indirect measurement of end-diastolic volume seems to be a better indicator of both preload and preload recruitable increases in cardiac output in response to fluid challenge.[13,22,24]

Table 1. Measured Hemodynamic Variables

Variable (abbreviation)	Unit	NormalRange
Systolic blood pressure (SBP)	Torr	100-140
Diastolic blood pressure (DBP)	Torr	60-90
Mean arterial pressure (MAP)	Torr	70-105
Pulmonary artery systolic pressure (PASP)	Torr	15-30
Pulmonary artery diastolic pressure (PADP)	Torr	4-12
Mean pulmonary artery pressure (MPAP)	Torr	9-16
Right ventricular systolic pressure (RVSP)	Torr	15-30
Right ventricular end diastolic pressure (RVEDP)	Torr	0-8
Central venous pressure (CVP)	Torr	0-8
Pulmonary artery occlusion pressure (PAOP)	Torr	2-12
Cardiac output (CO)	L/min	(Varies with size)
Stroke volume (SV)	mL/beat	(Varies with size)

Normal values for directly and indirectly measured hemodynamic variables.

Ventricular afterload is equally difficult to assess. Afterload is generally defined as the impedance to ejection from the left ventricle.[47,63] This means that left ventricular afterload is determined by aortic valve resistance, left ventricular compliance, aortic compliance, systemic vascular resistance, and the mass and viscosity of the blood. The variable which is most easily assessed and treated is the systemic vascular resistance. Since this value is calculated from the cardiac output, it must be indexed to body surface area in order to be interpreted. While there are many determinants of systemic vascular resistance index, isolated intravascular volume depletion in the absence of confounding medications and other pathophysiologic states (i.e., sepsis) is usually associated with an increase in systemic vascular resistance index.[55]

OXYGEN TRANSPORT AS AN ASSESSMENT OF INTRAVASCULAR VOLUME ADEQUACY

Oxygen Transport Terminology

Because of the uncertainty and the variability of individual patient responses to decreases in oxygen carrying capacity, physiologic indicators of the *adequacy* of oxygen delivery have been proposed. Unfortunately, oxygen transport terminology has become increasingly complex in the last several years.[65]

The components of oxygen transport may be assessed using both directly measured and calculated variables. The variables fall under two general categories: hemodynamics and oxygenation. The hemodynamic variables are those which are used to assess cardiac function and, in particular, those which affect cardiac output. Cardiac output is the product of heart rate and stroke volume and stroke volume is determined by the interaction between preload, afterload, and contractility (Tables 1 and 2).

Oxygen transport is assessed by combining oxygenation and hemodynamic variables (Table 3)

Table 2. Variables Derived from Hemodynamic Measurements

Variable (abbreviation)	Unit	Normal Range
Cardiac index (CI)	$L/min/m^2$	2.8-4.2
Stroke volume index (SVI)	$mL/beat/m^2$	30-65
Right ventricular ejection fraction (RVEF)	fraction	0.40-0.60
Right ventricular end-diastolic volume index (RVEDVI)	mL/m^2	60-100
Left ventricular stroke work index (LVSWI)	$g \cdot m/m^2$	43-61
Right ventricular stroke work index (RVSWI)	$g \cdot m/m^2$	7-12
Systemic vascular resistance index (SVRI)	$dyne \cdot sec \cdot cm^{-5}/m^2$	1600-2400
Pulmonary vascular resistance index (PVRI)	$dyne \cdot sec \cdot cm^{-5}/m^2$	250-430

Normal values for derived hemodynamic variables.

There is general agreement that oxygen delivery defines the volume of gaseous oxygen which is pumped from the left ventricle each minute. Oxygen delivery (DO_2) is therefore the product of cardiac output (or its index, CI) and arterial oxygen content (CaO_2). Normal oxygen delivery is about 600 $mL/min/m^2$.

The other side of the oxygen transport balance is oxygen consumption (VO_2). Oxygen consumption defines the volume of gaseous oxygen which is actually *used* by the body each minute. Oxygen consumption is a value which is calculated using the Fick equation. The Fick equation simply says that the volume of oxygen consumed is equal to the difference between the volume of oxygen delivered to the body minus the volume of oxygen returned to the heart. This is calculated by the classic equation of $VO_2 = C(a-v)O_2$ x CI. Normal oxygen consumption is about 140 $mL/min/m^2$.

Oxygen utilization defines the fraction of delivered oxygen which is actually consumed. Therefore, the oxygen utilization coefficient (OUC) is equal to VO_2/DO_2. The OUC is an indicator of the relative oxygen transport balance. The normal OUC ranges from about 0.2 to 0.3. Values greater than

Table 3. Variables Derived from Analysis of Gases

Variable (abbreviation)	Unit	Normal Range
Arterial oxygen tension (PaO_2)	Torr	70-100
Arterial oxygen saturation (SaO_2)	fraction	0.93-0.98
Arterial oxygen content (CaO_2)	mL/dL	16-22
Mixed venous oxygen tension (PvO_2)	Torr	36-42
Mixed venous oxygen saturation (SvO_2)	fraction	0.70-0.78
Mixed venous oxygen content (CvO_2)	mL/dL	12-17
Arterial-venous oxygen content difference ($C(a-v)O_2$)	mL/dL	3.5-5.5
Oxygen delivery index (DO_2)	$mL/min/m^2$	500-650
Oxygen consumption index (VO_2)	$mL/min/m^2$	110-150
Oxygen utilization coefficient (OUC)	fraction	0.22-0.30
Carbon dioxide production index (VCO_2)	$mL/min/m^2$	90-150
Respiratory quotient (RQ)	fraction	0.7-1.0
Pulmonary venous admixture (Qsp/Qt)	fraction	0.03-0.08

Normal values for measured and derived variables obtained by gas analysis.

0.35 indicate a severe stress upon oxygen delivery to adequately meet the oxygen consumption requirements of the patient.

Oxygen demand is a relatively new term which is used to define the volume of oxygen which is actually *needed* by the tissues to function aerobically.[43] At this time we have no technology available to measure actual oxygen demand. Therefore, we must rely on indirect indicators of the relationship between the demand for oxygen (what is needed) and the consumption of oxygen (what is used). When the demand for oxygen exceeds the consumption of oxygen, anaerobic metabolism must occur or the tissues will die. Therefore, markers of anaerobic metabolism, such as lactic acid concentration, serve to indicate that the demand for oxygen has exceeded the consumption of oxygen.[44]

The last term commonly used today to define oxygen transport is the oxygen uptake. Oxygen uptake defines the volume of gaseous oxygen which is removed from the patient's gas supply each minute. This value is what is commonly measured through indirect calorimetry on modern metabolic measurement carts. Oxygen uptake can differ from oxygen consumption and oxygen demand depending upon the patient's metabolic status and pulmonary status.

Monitoring Oxygen Transport Balance

Oxygen transport balance is clearly defined by the variables in the Fick equation. The balance of oxygen supply and demand is dependent upon the relative relationship between those factors which determine supply (cardiac index, hemoglobin concentration, and arterial oxygen saturation) and oxygen consumption (VO_2). Since these variables are related to one another by physical laws, the relationships are predictable and calculable.

For years mixed venous oxygen tension (PvO_2) has been used to help the clinician assess tissue oxygenation. It is clear that PvO_2 does not well define tissue oxygenation but yet is an important predictor of the likelihood of the development of anaerobic metabolism and associated mortality. In the early 1980s, technology became available to allow the continuous monitoring of mixed venous oxygen saturation by using fiberoptics embedded in the wall of a flow directed pulmonary artery catheter. Using three wave lengths of light, the relative fraction of oxyhemoglobin to total hemoglobin contained in red cells flowing past the end of the fiberoptic catheter could be determined. This fraction represents the mixed venous oxygen saturation (SvO_2).

It was initially believed that the SvO_2 would be closely related to cardiac output. It was disappointing to many early investigators to find that many other factors affecting oxygen supply and demand influenced SvO_2 so that it could not be reliably used as an indicator of cardiac output. When the Fick equation is solved for SvO_2, it becomes clear that SvO_2 is far more important than merely an indicator of cardiac output.[64] It is, in fact, an indicator of the relative balance between the supply and demand of oxygen:

$$SvO_2 = \frac{VO_2}{co \times Hb \times SaO_2} = 1 - \frac{VO_2}{DO_2} = 1 - OUC$$

The mixed venous oxygen saturation is therefore an indicator of the relative balance between oxygen supply and demand. It is a sensitive but nonspecific indicator that an imbalance has occurred. It does not define the nature of the imbalance or by itself give insights into the therapy which could be used to improve the oxygen transport balance. Rather, SvO_2 is the flow weighted average of the venous effluents from all perfused vascular beds. Therefore, it does not define the oxygen supply/demand adequacy of individual vascular beds but rather the entire body as a whole. Because of this, high flow, low extraction beds (such as the kidney) have greater impact on SvO_2 than do high extraction, low flow beds (such as the myocardium).

ASSESSMENT OF TRANSFUSION NEED

Oxygen transport variables are related to the consumption of oxygen by the tissues. Once the clinician comes to the understanding that the primary role of the cardiopulmonary system is to provide adequate oxygen for the tissues to function aerobically, it becomes obvious that a basic treatment principle is to maximize oxygen consumption. That is to say that the use of oxygen by the patient should be allowed to rise to whatever level is required to meet the demand for oxygen created by the tissues. Since the demand for oxygen cannot yet be measured directly, we must allow the consumption (use) to reach maximum values but at the same time not place the patient in a situation of excessive demand for oxygen (agitation, fever,

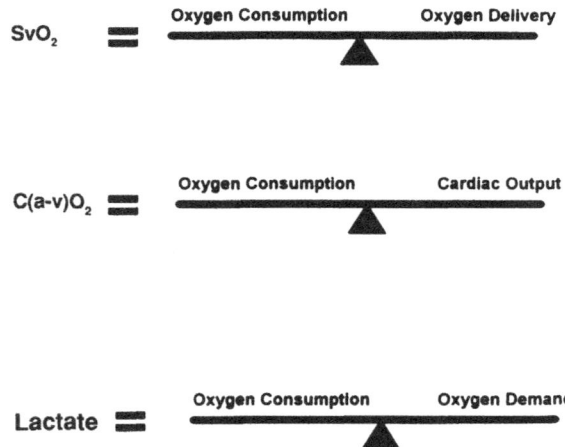

Figure 2. The three critical balances. Three oxygen transport balances are often assessed in critically ill postoperative patients. Each of the balances assess the relationship between oxygen consumption and other variables. The balance between oxygen consumption and oxygen delivery is assessed by measuring the mixed venous oxygen saturation (SvO_2 or the oxygen utilization coefficient (extraction ratio, VO_2/DO_2). The balance between oxygen consumption and cardiac output is determined by the Fick equation to be equal to the arterial-venous oxygen content difference, $C(a-v)O_2$. The balance between oxygen demand (the volume needed to function aerobically) and oxygen consumption (the volume actually used) is reflected by the arterial lactate level. When oxygen demand exceeds oxygen consumption, excess lactate appears.

seizures, shivering, pain, etc.). When use of oxygen (consumption) equals the demand for oxygen the patient's oxygen transport needs are met.

Three critical balances must be assessed (Figure 2). The balance between oxygen delivery and consumption is assessed by measuring the SvO_2. When arterial oxygenation is adequate ($SaO_2 > 0.90$), the SvO_2 is inversely related to the oxygen utilization coefficient (OUC). The OUC quantitates the fraction of delivered oxygen which is consumed and, therefore, defines the oxygen-supply demand balance.

The balance between oxygen consumption and total blood flow must be assessed next. If SvO_2 is < 0.60-0.65, the delivery of oxygen may be inadequate for the consumption needed to maintain optimal cellular function. Since the decrease in SvO_2 is sensitive but not specific for any individual cause for the imbalance (SaO_2, hemoglobin concentration, cardiac output, or VO_2), further assessment is necessary. The second critical balance is between cardiac output and VO_2. The $C(a-v)O_2$ defines this balance.

The third critical balance is between the consumption (use) of oxygen and the demand (need) created by the tissues. When the need for oxygen exceeds the actual use, the tissues must switch to inefficient anaerobic pathways of metabolism or they will have no energy production at all and will die. While anaerobic energy production is better than no energy production, it cannot continue indefinitely. Short term anaerobic metabolism saves the patient from immediate death in times of severe tissue hypoxia but is one of the first steps into the spiraling cycle of organ dysfunction, failure, and death. Arterial (or mixed venous) lactate levels are one of the most clinically useful indicators of anaerobic metabolism.

Thus, there are two types of indicators for transfusion of red blood cells in anemic, critically ill patients: clinical and physiologic. The clinical indications include tachycardia, hypotension, oliguria, cutaneous hypoperfusion, and alterations in mental status not related to other causes. The physiologic indicators of significant impairment of oxygen transport include $SvO_2 < 0.60$ (or $PvO_2 < 30$ mm Hg), OUC > 0.35, $DO_2 < 450$ mL/min/m^2, $C(a-v)O_2 > 5.5$ mL/dL and a lactic acid level > 2.5 mmol/dL. When the hemoglobin concentration falls below acceptable values these indicators suggest potential benefit from transfusion. The trick is knowing the acceptable hemoglobin concentration. Clearly, transfusing red cells when the hemoglobin is > 14-15 g/dL is virtually *never* of value in improving oxygen transport. On the other hand, transfusing when the oxygen transport indices suggest doing so is almost always of value when the hemoglobin is < 8 g/dL. Clinical experience (but not scientific data) suggests that oxygen transport balance *usually* improves with transfusion when the hemoglobin is 8-11 g/dL. The same experience suggests that in *some* patients with inadequate oxygen transport, transfusion improves tissue oxygenation when the hemoglobin concentration is 11-13 g/dL. Since the early 1980s the adequacy of cardiac output has generally been defined in terms of oxygen transport variables. These include the delivery of oxygen from the left ventricle, the consumption of oxygen by the peripheral tissues and the ratio of these two variables, the oxygen utilization coefficient. Intravascular volume depletion usually results in a compromise in oxygen delivery to the tissue. Severe reductions in oxygen delivery may result in a flow limitation of oxygen consumption which when unchecked, may result in anaerobic metabolism, further shock, and death of the patient.[34,36]

The addition of mixed venous oximetry to the flow-directed pulmonary artery catheter has allowed on-line assessment of these oxygen transport indices.[64] A decrease in mixed venous oxygen saturation is a sensitive but non-specific indicator of global oxygen transport imbalance. A decrease in mixed venous oxygen saturation indicates an increase in the oxygen utilization coefficient (oxygen extraction ratio) which means that a greater fraction of delivered oxygen is being consumed. Mixed venous oxygen saturation is also used in the calculation of the arterial-venous oxygen content difference $[C(a-v)O_2]$ which is an indicator of the adequacy of cardiac output in meeting tissue oxygen consumption. An increase in $C(a-v)O_2$ indicates greater extraction of oxygen by the tissue to maintain the necessary oxygen consumption (Figure 2). When hemodynamic measurements indicate that reduced preload may be at least partially responsible for an impairment in oxygen transport, a volume challenge intended to optimize preload thus improving cardiac output and oxygen delivery seems warranted.[5,23,45]

Treatment with preload augmentation to reach an optimal oxygen delivery value or to achieve a level of oxygen consumption that is independent of delivery may prove to be desirable therapeutic end-points.[80,96] This is most efficiently achieved by transfusing red cells but, when hemoglobin concentration has been optimized, other fluids may be used.

The last indicator of inadequate oxygen transport is the presence of significant lactic acidosis. This is generally considered to be a marker that anaerobic metabolism has occurred and that, at least for a period of time, the demand for oxygen at the tissue level has exceeded the actual use of oxygen by the tissue. The clearance of lactate and the accompanying metabolic acidosis generally indicates an improvement in oxygen transport balance.[44,74] The fluid challenge may be an important diagnostic and therapeutic maneuver in patients with lactic acidosis unexplained by other reasons.[26]

CLINICAL RECOMMENDATIONS

Transfusion of blood and blood products is a major decision in many critically ill patients. The trigger for transfusion varies with the severity of illness and is not merely an arbitrary value of hemoglobin concentration. Probably the best rule is to maintain an adequate circulating blood volume and oxygen transport balance so that organ perfusion is optimized. When hemoglobin concentration is low or the patient is actively bleeding or suspected to be bleeding, blood is currently the best solution to depleted intravascular volume. By resuscitating the shock state, capillary membrane function will be maintained and the need for large volumes of crystalloid solutions will be reduced. Maintaining good end-organ function is the best indicator of the adequacy of intravascular volume. When the end-organ function is compromised or is difficult to monitor, invasive assessment of oxygen transport function may be necessary to optimize cardio-pulmonary performance. Development of impaired oxygen delivery or oxygen consumption, increased oxygen utilization, or lactic acidosis in an anemic patient should prompt transfusion of blood products.

The priorities for perioperative fluid management continue to be replacement of: 1) red cell mass, 2) coagulation factors in the patient at high risk for bleeding, 3) intravascular volume and, 4) maintenance of adequate interstitial volume. A physiologic approach to transfusion based on a careful assessment of oxygen transport determined by the patient and goal-directed administration of fluids and blood products to predetermined physiologic end-points can be effective in reducing postoperative organ system dysfunction and failure.

REFERENCES

1. Aach RD, Kahn RA: Post-transfusion hepatitis: current perspectives. Ann Intern Med 1980;92:539.
2. Agarwal N, Murphy JG, Cayten CG, Stahl WM: Blood transfusion increases the risk of infection after trauma. Arch Surg 1993;128:171-177.
3. Alexander JW: Transfusion-induced immunomodulation and infection. Transfusion 1991;31:195-196.
4. Auler JOC, Pereira MHC, Gomide-Araral RV, et al: Hemodynamic effects of hypertonic sodium chloride during surgical treatment of aortic aneurysms. Surgery 1987;101:594.
5. Barone JE, Snyder AB: Treatment strategies in shock: Use of oxygen transport measurements. Heart Lung 1991;20:81.
6. Bauer M, Marzi I, Ziegenfu BT, et al: Comparative effects of crystalloid and small volume hypertonic hyperoncotic fluid resuscitation on hepatic microcirculation after hemorrhagic shock. Cir Shock 1993;40:187-193.
7. Baxter CR, Zedlitz WH, Shires GT: High-output acute renal failure complicating traumatic injury. J Trauma 1964;4:467.
8. Bisonni RS, Holtgrave DR, Lawler R, et al: Colloids versus crystalloids in fluid resuscitation: An analysis of randomized controlled trials. J Fam Pract 1991;32:387.
9. Bland JHL, Laver MB, Lowenstein E: Vasodilator effect of commercial 5% plasma protein fraction solutions. JAMA 1973;224:1721.
10. Canizaro PC, Prager MD, Shires GT: The infusion of Ringer's lactate solution during shock. Am J Surg 1971;122:494.
11. Carrico CJ, Canizaro PC, Shires T: Fluid resuscitation following injury: rationale for the use of balanced salt solutions. Crit Care Med 1976;4:46-54.
12. Chaudry IH, Ayala A, Wolfgang E, Stephan R: Hemorrhage and resuscitation; Immunological aspects. Amer Physiological Soc 1990;R663-R678.
13. Cheatham ML, Chang MC, Eddy VA, Safcsak K, Nelson LD: Right ventricular end-diastolic volume index and pulmonary artery occlusion. Chest 1993;104(2):78S.
14. Cogbill TH, Moore EE, Dunn EL, et al: Coagulation changes after albumin resuscitation. Crit Care Med 1981;9:22.
15. Collins JA: Problems associated with the massive transfusion of stored blood. Surgery 1974;75:274.
16. Cone JB, Wallce BH, Caldwell FT Jr, et al: Beneficial effects of a hypertonic solution for resuscitation in the presence of acute hemorrhage. Am J Surg 1987;154:585.
17. Counts RB, Haisch C, Simon TL, et al: Hemostasis in massively transfused trauma patients. Ann Surg 1979;7:91-98.
18. Cue JI, Peyton JC, Malangoni MA: Does blood transfusion or hemorrhagic shock induce immunosuppression? J Trauma 1992;32:613-617.
19. Czer LSC, Shoemaker WC: Optimal hematocrit value in critically ill postoperative patients. Surg Gynecol Obstet 1978;147:363.
20. D'Angio R, Orlando R: Fluid resuscitation: Colloid versus crystalloid. Connecticut Med 1986;50:689-691.
21. Dahn MS, Lucas CE, Ledgerwood AM, et al: Negative inotropic effect of albumin resuscitation for shock. Surgery 1979;86:235.

22. Diebel LN, Wilson RF, Taggett MG, et al: End-diastolic volume: A better indicator of preload in the critically ill. Arch Surg 1992;127:817.
23. Domsky MF, Wilson RF: Hemodynamic resuscitation. Crit Care Clin 1993;10:715-726.
24. Eddy VA, Chang MC, Cheatham ML, Safcsak K, Nelson LD: Reevaluation of the bedside approach to preload assessment. Chest 1993;104:73S.
25. Edna TH, Bjerkeset T: Association between blood transfusion and infection in injured patients. J Trauma 1992;33:659-661.
26. Falk JL, Rackow EC, Leavy J, et al: Delayed lactate clearance in patients surviving circulatory shock. Acute Care 1985;11:212.
27. Fortune JB, Feustel PJ, Saifi J, et al: Influence of hematocrit on cardiopulmonary function after acute hemorrhage. J Trauma 1987;27:243-249.
28. Freshman SP, Battistella FD, Matteucci M, et al: Hypertonic saline (7.5%) versus mannitol: A comparison for treatment of acute head injuries. J Trauma 1993;35:344-348.
29. Gallagher TJ, Banner MJ, Barnes PA: Large volume crystalloid resuscitation does not increase extravascular lung water. Anesth Analg 1985;64:323.
30. Gann DS, Carlson DE, Byrnes GJ, Pirkle JC Jr, and Allen-Rowlands CS: Role of solute in the early restitution of blood volume after hemorrhage. Surgery 1983;94:439.
31. Glover JL, Broadie TA: Autotransfusion in trauma. Crit Care Quarterly 1983;6:33-43.
32. Graves TA, Cioffi WG, et al: Relationship of transfusion and infection in a burn population. J Trauma 1989;29:948-954.
33. Gross D, Landau EH, Klin B, et al: Treatment of uncontrolled hemorrhagic shock with hypertonic saline solution. Surg Gynecol Obstet 1990;170:106.
34. Hankeln K, Radel C, Becz M, et al: Comparison of hydroxy-ethyl starch and lactated Ringer's solution on hemodynamics and oxygen transport in critically ill patients in prospective crossover studies. Crit Care Med 1989;17:133.
35. Harrigan C, Lucas CE, Ledgerwood AM, et al: Serial changes in primary hemostasis after massive transfusion. Surgery 1985;98:836-843.
36. Haupt MT, Gilbert EM, Carlson RW: Fluid loading increases oxygen consumption in septic patients with lactic acidosis. Am Rev Respir Dis 1985;131:912.
37. Heimbach DM: Hemostasis in massively transfused trauma patients. In: Fresh Frozen Plasma: Indicators and risks. NIH Consensus Development Conference, Bethesda, MD, 1984:38-39.
38. Hewson JR, Neame PB, Kumar N, et al: Coagulopathy related to dilution and hypotension during massive transfusion. Crit Care Med 1985;13:387-391.
39. Holcroft JW, Trunkey DD: Pulmonary extravasation of albumin during and after hemorrhagic shock in baboons. J Surg Res 1975;18:91.
40. Holcroft JW, Trunkey DD: Extravascular lung water following hemorrhagic shock in the baboon: Comparison between resuscitation with Ringer's lactate and plasmanate. Ann Surg 1974;180:408-417.
41. Imm A, Carlson RW: Fluid resuscitation in circulatory shock. Crit Care Clin 1993;9:313-333.
42. Johnson SD, Lucas CE, Gerrick SJ, et al: Altered coagulation after albumin supplements for treatment of oligemic shock. Arch Surg 1979;114:379-383.
43. Kandel G, Aberman A: Mixed venous oxygen saturation: Its role in the assessment of the critically ill patient. Arch Int Med 1983;143:1400-1402.
44. Kasnitz P, Druger GL, Yorra F, Simmons DH. Mixed venous oxygen tension and hyperlactatemia: Survival in severe cardiopulmonary disease. JAMA 1976;236:570-574.
45. Komatsu T, Shibutani K, Okamoto K, et al: Critical level of oxygen delivery after cardiopulmonary bypass. Crit Care Med 1987;15:194.
46. Kovalik SG, Ledgerwood AM, Lucas CE, et al: The cardiac effect of altered calcium homeostasis after albumin resuscitation. J Trauma 1981;21:275.
47. Lappas DG, Fahmy NR: The heart. In: Burke JF (Ed): Surgical Physiology. Saunders, Philadelphia, PA, 1983:476-496.
48. Lucas CE, Ledgerwood AM, Mammon EF: Altered coagulation protein content after varied resuscitation regimens. J Trauma 1982;22:1.
49. Lucas CE, Ledgerwood A, Mammon EF: Altered coagulation protein content after albumin resuscitation. Ann Surg 1982;196:198-202.

50. Lucas CE, Ledgerwood AM, Higgins RE, et al: Impaired pulmonary function after albumin resuscitation from shock. J Trauma 1980;20:446.

51. Lucas CE, Bouwman DL, Ledgerwood AM, Higgins R. Differential serum protein changes following supplemental albumin resuscitation for hypovolemic shock. J Trauma 1980;20:47.

52. Lucas CE, Weaver D. Higgins RF, Ledgerwood AM, et al. Effects of albumin versus non-albumin resuscitation on plasma volume and renal excretory function. J Trauma 1978;18:564.

53. Martin DJ, Lucas, CE, Ledgerwood AM, et al: Fresh frozen plasma supplement to massive red blood cell transfusion. Ann Surg 1985;202:505-510.

54. Booth FVMcL: Fluid resuscitation of the critically ill: Monitoring in Resuscitation. Crit Care Clin 1992;8:455.

55. Mellander S, Johannson B: Control of resistance, exchange, and capacitance functions in the peripheral circulation. Pharmacol Rev 1968;20:117.

56. Metildi LA, Shackford SR, Virgilio RW, et al: Crystalloid versus colloid in fluid resuscitation of patients with severe pulmonary insufficiency. Surg Gynecol Obstet 1984;158:207.

57. Mezrow CK, Bergstein I, Tartter PI: Postoperative infections following autologous and homologous blood transfusions. Transfusion 1992;32:27-30.

58. Miller RD: Medical intelligence: Complications of massive blood transfusions, Anesth 1973;39:82-93.

59. Monafo WW, Halverson JD, Schechtman K: The role of concentrated sodium solutions in the resuscitation of patients with severe burns. Surgery 1984;95:129.

60. Moss GS: An argument in favor of electrolyte solution for early resuscitation. Surg Clin North Am 1972;52:3.

61. Moylan JA, Reckler JM, Mason AD: Resuscitation with hypertonic lactate saline in thermal injury. Am J Surg 1973;125:580.

62. Myhre B: Fatalities from blood transfusion. JAMA 1980;244:1333-1335.

63. Nelson LD, Snyder JV: Technical problems in data acquisition. In: Marshall DK, Kelly KM (Eds): Oxygen transport in the critically ill. Year Book Medical Publishers, Inc., Chicago, IL, 1987:205-234.

64. Nelson LD: Continuous venous oximetry in surgical patients. Ann Surg 1986;2Q3:329.

65. Nelson LD: Assessment of oxygenation: Oxygenation indices. Respir Care 38:631-645, 1993.

66. Opelz G, Sengar DPS, Mickey MR, Terasaki P: Effect of blood transfusions on subsequent kidney transplants. Transplant Proc 1973;5:253-9.

67. Peters RM, Shackford SR, Hogan JS, et al: Comparison of isotonic and hypertonic fluids in resuscitation from hypovolemic shock. Surg Gynecol Obstet 1986;163:219.

68. Phillips TF, Soulier G, Wilson RF: Outcome of massive transfusion exceeding two blood volumes in trauma and emergency surgery. J Trauma 1987;27:903-910.

69. Prough DS, Johnson JC, Poole GV, et al: Effects on intracranial pressure of resuscitation from hemorrhagic shock with hypertonic saline versus lactated Ringer's solution. Crit Care Med 1985;13:407.

70. Rackow EC, Falk JL, Fein IA, et al: Fluid resuscitation in circulatory shock: A comparison of the cardiorespiratory effects of albumin, hetastarch and saline solutions in patients with hypovolemic and septic shock. Crit Care Med 1983;11:839-850.

71. Reed RL II, Ciavarella D, et al: Prophylactic platelet administration during massive transfusion. Ann Surgery 1986;203:40-48.

72. Reuse C, Vincent JL, Pinsky MR: Measurements of right ventricular volumes during fluid challenge. Chest 1990;98:1450.

73. Rosemurgery AS, Hart MB, Murphy CG, et al: Infection after injury. Amer Surgeon 1992;58:104-107.

74. Rutherford EJ, Morris JA, Reed GW, et al: Base deficit stratifies mortality and determines therapy. J Trauma 1992;33:417-423.

75. Schaeffer RC, Reniewicz RA, Chilton SM, et al: Effects of colloid or crystalloid solutions on edemagenesis in normal and thrombomicroembolized lungs. Crit Care Med 1987;15:1110-1115.

76. Shires GT, Carrico CT, Cohn D: The role of extracellular fluid in shock. Int Anaesth Clin 1964;2:435.

77. Shires GT, Cunningham JN, Baker CRF, Reeder SF, Illner H, Wagner IY, Maher J: Alterations in cellular membrane function during hemorrhagic shock in primates. Ann Surg 1972;176:288.

78. Shires T, Cohn D, Carrico J, et al: Fluid therapy in hemorrhagic shock. Arch Surg 1964;88:688.

79. Shoemaker WC, Appel PL, Kram HB, et al: Prospective trial of supranormal values of survivors as therapeutic goals in high-risk surgical patients. Chest 1988;94:1176-1186.

80. Shoemaker WC: A new approach to physiology, monitoring, and therapy of shock states. World J Surg 1987;11:133.

81. Siegel DC, Cochin A, Geocaris T, et al: Effects of saline and colloid resuscitation on renal function. Ann Surg 1973;177:51-57.

82. Stahl WM: Crystalloid versus colloid resuscitation. Trauma Quarterly 1985;5:15-23.

83. Sutin KM, Ruskin KJ, Kaufman BS: Intravenous fluid therapy in neurologic injury. Crit Care Clin 1992;8:367-408.

84. Todd MH, Tommasino C, Moore S: Cerebral effects of isovolemic hemodilution with a hypertonic saline solution. J Neurosurg 1985;63:944.

85. Valeri CR, Feingold H, et al: Hypothermia-induced reversible platelet dysfunction. Ann Surg 1987;205:175-181.

86. Vassar MJ, Fischer RP, O'Brien PE, et al: A multicenter trial for resuscitation of injured patients with 7.5% sodium chloride. Arch Surg 1993;128:1003-1013.

87. Vassar MJ, Perry CA, Holcroft JW: Prehospital resuscitation of hypotensive trauma patients with 7.5% NaCl versus 7.5% NaCl with added dextran: A controlled trial. J Trauma 1993;34:622-633.

88. Velanovich V: Crystalloid versus colloid fluid resuscitation: A meta-analysis of mortality. Surgery 1989;105:65-71.

89. Vincent JL: Plugging the leaks: New insight into synthetic colloids. Crit Care Med 1991;19:316.

90. Virgilio RW, Rice CL, Smith DE, et al: Crystalloid vs colloid resuscitation: Is one better? Surgery 1979;85:129.

91. Watkins GM, Glover JL, Greenburg AG, Friedman BA: Panel: "Present use of blood and blood products". J Trauma 1981;21:1005-1012.

92. Weaver DW, Ledgerwood AM, Lucas CE, et al: Pulmonary effects of albumin resuscitation for severe hypovolemic shock. Arch Surg 1978;113:387.

93. Wilson RF: Complications of massive transfusions. Surgical Rounds 1981;8:47-54.

94. Wu HS, Little AG: Perioperative blood transfusions and cancer recurrence. J Clin Oncol 1988;6:1348-54.

95. Yeston NS, Niehoff JM, Dennis RC: Transfusion therapy. In: Civetta JM, Taylor RW, Kirby RR (Eds) Critical Care, Second Ed. Lippincott, Philadelphia, PA, 1992:427-443.

96. Yu M, Levy MM, Smith P, et al: Effect of maximizing oxygen delivery on morbidity and mortality rates in critically ill patients: A prospective randomized, controlled trial. Crit Care Med 1993;21:830-838.

PREOPERATIVE AUTOLOGOUS BLOOD DONATION

Lawrence T. Goodnough, MD

Washington University School of Medicine
Barnes Hospital
St. Louis, Missouri

Interest in blood conservation interventions has been stimulated by recent emphasis on issues of blood safety, blood inventory, and alternatives to allogeneic (from an anonymous, volunteer donor) blood transfusion.[1] One of these alternatives is "no transfusion: a lowering of the transfusion-trigger", that hematocrit (Hct) level at which physicians empirically decide to transfuse.[2] Recent studies have suggested that the transfusion-trigger hematocrit has been lowered by increasingly conservative transfusion practice for patients undergoing elective blood transfusion in settings such as elective surgery.[3-5]

A second alternative to allogeneic blood transfusion is blood transfusion from a designated (known to the blood transfusion recipient) donor; this is a controversial transfusion practice, since current evidence suggests that directed blood transfusions are no safer, and in fact may be less safe, than allogeneic blood.[6-9] Recent studies have indicated that designated donation does not minimize allogeneic blood transfusion in patients undergoing elective orthopaedic surgery;[10] furthermore, directed donor programs may adversely affect participation in autologous donation programs.[11]

A third alternative to allogeneic blood is autologous blood transfusion. A progressive evolution of blood conservation techniques including intraoperative and/or postoperative salvage and reinfusion has occurred in open heart surgical patients. National guidelines published recently have emphasized that in elective settings in which a decision to transfuse is made, the preferred alternative is autologous blood.[12,13] Autologous blood has several advantages: autologous blood is the safest blood,[14] it adds to the regional blood inventory,[15] and it reinforces conservative transfusion practice.[4] Autologous blood can be procured in the surgical setting by utilizing one or more conservation interventions: preoperative autologous blood donation, acute preoperative hemodilution, and perioperative autologous blood salvage. For transfusion settings such as elective surgery, preoperative autologous blood donation represents an attractive alternative to allogeneic blood

Critical Issues in Surgery, Edited by A. C. Cernaianu et al.
Plenum Press, New York, 1995

transfusion. This previously underutilized practice[16] has become a standard of care in several elective surgical procedures,[17] resulting in a significant increase in the percentage of blood collected nationally that is autologous.[18] Potential candidates for autologous blood donation prior to elective surgery include any patient scheduled for a procedure for whom blood type and crossmatch is requested[19] indicating a likelihood of requiring blood transfusion according to a maximum surgical blood ordering schedule.[20] Underutilization of autologous donation before elective surgery has been improved with coordinated programs involving the regional blood center, the hospital blood bank, information services, and physicians. Using this approach studies have found that for autologous blood donors, 9 percent of all patients undergoing all elective surgery,[21] 17 percent of patients undergoing orthopaedic surgery,[3] and from 9 to 15 percent of patients undergoing radical prostatectomy,[22-24] subsequently received allogeneic blood.

The relationship between autologous blood ordering, blood collection, and subsequent exposure to allogeneic blood was examined in a recent study of 263 orthopaedic surgical patients.[25] Surgeons followed the same autologous blood ordering guidelines for orthopaedic procedures as were established for ordering crossmatched allogeneic blood.[26] The schedule of donations was determined by the preoperative donation time interval (date of first phlebotomy until date of surgery) and the number of autologous blood units requested. A previous analysis reported that a mean of 3 autologous blood units was requested for orthopaedic patients over an average collection period of 22 days, so that standard phlebotomy practice was to schedule one donation approximately every 7 days.[27] Eighty-four (32 percent) of 263 patients were unable to store the number of autologous blood units requested, of which 70 (83 percent) were female patients. Twenty-three (27 percent) of 84 patients in this blood procurement cohort subsequently received allogeneic blood. Of these, only 3 (2 percent) of 146 patients asked to donate ≤3 units received allogeneic blood, compared to 20 (17 percent) of 116 patients asked to donate ≥4 units (p <0.01).

One important factor that contributes to the likelihood of allogeneic blood exposure in this setting is the *transfusion trigger*. Transfusion practices have an important role in determining the *success* or *failure* of many blood conservation interventions.[28] A previous analysis indicated that 25 percent of autologous donors and 11 percent of non-autologous donors could be identified who were transfused with blood in excess of needs.[29]

Another factor that determines the risk of subsequent allogeneic blood transfusion is the presence of anemia at first blood donation, especially in patients asked to predonate ≥4 autologous units.[25,27] The prevalence of allogeneic blood exposure related to blood procurement in anemic patients asked to donate ≥4 units in two studies was 35 percent (13 of 37 patients),[30] and 40 percent (23 of 58 patients),[31] indicating the need for innovative approaches in blood conservation in this population.

In one clinical trial,[32] patients were subjected to aggressive autologous phlebotomy according to standards of the American Association of Blood Banks (procurement goal of 6 units in 3 weeks as long as Hct ≥33 percent).[33] As illustrated in figure 1, such an approach generated the production and replacement of an additional red blood cell volume equivalent to nearly 3 (allogeneic) blood units.[34]

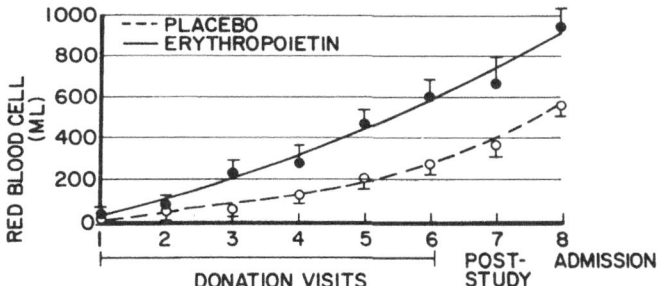

Figure 1. Red blood cell (RBC) production during autologous blood donation, in 23 placebo (open circles) and 21 erythropoietin (closed circles) treated patients. Data points represent calculated RBC production from donation visits 1 through 6, post-study visit, and hospital admission. From Goodnough LT, et al: Transfusion 1992;32:441-445.

The addition of recombinant human erythropoietin therapy (EPO) generated the equivalent of an additional 2 blood units, or nearly 5 total. While this approach can reduce the prevalence of subsequent allogeneic blood exposure in anemic patients from the 35-40 percent prevalence noted in the above studies to less than 20 percent,[35] aggressive autologous blood procurement is associated with higher costs, lower cost-effectiveness, and wastage of autologous blood.[24,36] Alternative and more cost-effective strategies for autologous blood procurement, such as acute preoperative hemodilution, are currently being investigated.[37] Targeting surgical procedures for which autologous blood donation is useful and should be promoted, and those procedures for which it is unnecessary and should be discouraged, should enhance its cost effectiveness.[35,36,38,39] A summary of such surgical procedures is shown in Table 1.

The same approach should be taken with blood conservation strategies.[40] A recent clinical trial found no role for EPO therapy in orthopaedic surgical patients who were not anemic (Hct >39 percent) at first donation of autologous blood.[41] However, a subsequent study in patients who were anemic (Hct ≤39 percent) at first donation showed a reduction in allogeneic blood exposure in patients treated with EPO, especially in females and in patients whose initial donation Hct level was <37 percent.[35] Thus, sub-

Table 1. Surgical Procedures Which May or May Not Benefit from Autologous Blood Predonation

"High" (5 percent) likelihood	"Low" (<5 percent) likelihood
Total joint orthopedic surgery	Vaginal hysterectomy
Complex spine surgery	Vaginal childbirth
Cardiac surgery	Caesarian section
Radical Prostatectomy	Cholecystectomy
Abdominal hysterectomy	Transurethral resection of the prostate
Vascular graft surgery	
Bone marrow harvest	
Mastectomy	
Colorectal surgery	
Craniotomy	

groups of patients can be identified who would benefit from this therapy, such as anemic patients, females and pediatric patients with smaller circulating red blood cell volumes.[32]

Many issues remain in need of definition for the use of erythropoietin therapy in the surgical setting. First, mobilization of iron stores and/or iron deficiency may limit the response to EPO through iron-restricted erythropoiesis. This has been analyzed for non-anemic autologous blood donors undergoing elective orthopaedic surgery, in which premenopausal females treated with EPO were demonstrated to need oral iron supplementation.[42] Additionally, for autologous blood donors who are anemic at the time of the first unit of blood donated, approximately one third of such patients are iron-depleted and require iron supplementation.[43] A recent study suggests that even with oral iron supplementation, autologous blood donors treated with EPO may have functional iron deficiency.[44] Alternative forms of oral or intravenous iron supplementation[45] may be needed in order to optimize the erythropoietic response to EPO therapy.

In addition, questions of optimal dose, route, and interval of administration for erythropoietin therapy in the surgical setting have yet to be established. Each of these issues is important in determining the cost-effectiveness of EPO therapy. Subcutaneous administration may be superior to an intravenous route, in that lower doses of EPO may be sufficient for the desired effect on erythropoiesis.[46,47] Data published to date indicate that the response to EPO administered intravenously occurs within 3.5 days [32] and that the equivalent of one blood unit (200 mL)[48] is produced within 7 days.[34] The EPO dosage (600 u/kg iv q3 days x 2) for a 70 kg patient to achieve this effect would total 84,000 units; at current prices of $0.01/unit,[49] the cost of EPO therapy to produce the equivalent of one blood unit can be estimated to be approximately $840. This can be compared to costs to patients for procurement of an autologous blood unit, ranging from $60 to $233 (mean $119) among 18 tertiary care institutions.[50] Alternative routes of administration and iron supplementation may significantly improve the cost-benefit ratio of EPO therapy. Recent reports of the cost-effectiveness of preoperative autologous blood donation [24,36,51] emphasize that blood conservation interventions, including pharmacologic agents, will be scrutinized and held accountable for their costs as well as by their benefits.

Finally, the prevalence of serious adverse concomitant events in patients treated with EPO needs to be monitored carefully and compared to untreated control groups. The prevalence of thrombotic events reported in an initial trial in dialysis patients[52] and in subsequent placebo-controlled trials in patients with chronic renal insufficiency[53,54] suggests that the interrelationship between hematocrit level, blood viscosity, and peripheral vascular resistance is important for thrombotic events in this setting.[55] Two studies of orthopaedic surgical patients without renal insufficiency who underwent aggressive autologous blood phlebotomy, with or without EPO therapy, reported thromboembolic events in two (one placebo, one EPO treated) of 47 patients[32] and two (one placebo, one EPO treated) of 116 patients;[41] the overall prevalence of four (2.4 percent) of 163 patients compares favorably to the prevalence of such events reported in patients who undergo orthopaedic joint replacement surgery.[56] Clinical trials in progress will provide additional information on the prevalence of such events in the perisurgical setting.[57]

Table 2. Guidelines for Recombinant Human Erythropoietin Therapy

I. Currently Approved Indications:
Anemia* in chronic renal failure (creat $\geq$ 1.8 mg percent)
Anemia with human immunodeficiency viral (HIV) infection undergoing treatment with zidovudine
Anemia in cancer patients undergoing chemotherapy
II. Indications Under Investigation
Anemia in chronic disease including rheumatoid arthritis
Autologous blood donation
Surgical blood loss
Bone marrow transplantation
Anemia of prematurity
Myelodysplastic syndromes
Sickle cell anemia
III. Current Contraindications
Patients in whom therapy will result in polycythemia
Patients with uncontrolled hypertension

*Anemia is defined as a reduced patient red cell volume, for which a blood transfusion is anticipated or needed.
From Goodnough LT et al.[58].

A summary of the current guidelines and indications for EPO therapy have been published recently.[58] The use of EPO in patients with surgical anemia should be restricted to clinical settings in which avoidance of blood transfusion has been demonstrated (Table 2).

Prudent use of EPO in patients at risk for surgical blood loss suggests that therapy should be linked to ongoing blood losses in order to avoid potential complications related to polycythemia and hypervicosity. The use of this agent to correct preoperative anemia should ideally be coupled with autologous blood procurement not only for these safety concerns, but to enhance the effectiveness of this therapy in reducing perisurgical allogeneic blood transfusions. For example, most blood transfusion support in coronary artery bypass surgery and orthopedic surgery is given on the day of operation and could be best avoided if autologous blood were available preoperatively.[59,60] Clinical trials which use allogeneic blood exposure as outcome are currently in progress in a variety of settings in order to demonstrate this.[57] Until these clinical trials are completed and published, the role of erythropoietin therapy in surgical anemia remains investigational.

REFERENCES

1. Goodnough LT, Shuck J: Blood tansfusion in elective surgery: review of risks, options, and informed consent. Am J Surg 1990;159:602-609.
2. Friedman BA, Burns TL, Schork MA: An analysis of blood transfusion of surgical patients by sex: A quest for the transfusion trigger. Transfusion 1980;20:179-188.
3. Goodnough LT, Shaffron D, Marcus RE: Impact of preoperative autologous blood donation in elective orthopaedic surgery. Vox Sang 1990;59:65-69.

4. Wasman J, Goodnough LT: Effect of autologous blood donation for elective surgery on physician transfusion behavior: a matched, controlled study. JAMA 1987;258:3135-3137.

5. Welch HG, Meehan KR, Goodnough LT: Prudent strategies for elective red blood cell transfusion. Ann Int Med 1992;116:393-402.

6. Goldfinger D: Directed Blood donations: Pro. Transfusion 1989;29:70-74.

7. Page PL: Directed blood donations: Con. Transfusion 1989;29:65-69.

8. Cordell RR, Yacon VA, Gigahn-Haskel Z, et al: Experience with 11,916 designated donors. Transfusion 1986;26:484-486.

9. Kruskall MS, Umlas J: Acquired immunodeficiency syndrome and directed blood donations. A dilemma for American medicine. Arch Surg 1988;123:23-25.

10. Goodnough LT: Predeposit of designated blood does not protect against homologous blood exposure in patients who predeposit autologous blood for elective surgery. Am J Clin Path 1989;92:484487.

11. Chambers LA, Kruskall MS, Leonard SS, Ellis AM: Directed donor programs may adversely affect autologous blood participation. Transfusion 1990;30:246-248.

12. National Institutes of Health Consensus Conferences: Perioperative red blood cell transfusion. JAMA 1988;260:2700-2703.

13. American College of Physicians: Practice strategies for elective red blood cell transfusion. Ann Intern Med 1992;116:403-406.

14. Surgenor DM: The patient's blood is the safest blood. N Engl J Med 1987;316:542-520.

15. Haugen K, Hill E: Large scale autologous blood program in a community hospital. JAMA 1987;257:1211-1214.

16. Toy PTCY, Strauss R, Stehling L, et al: Predeposit autologous blood for elective surgery: a multicenter study. NEJM 1987;316:517-520.

17. Kruskall MS, Glazer EE, Leonard SS, et al: Utilization and effectiveness of a hospital autologous preoperative blood donor program. Transfusion 1986;26:335-340.

18. Surgenor DM, Wallace EL, Hae SH, Chapman RH: Collection and transfusion of blood in the United States, 1982-1988. N Engl J Med 1990;332:1646-1651.

19. National Blood Resource Education Program Expert Panel. The Use of Autologous Blood. JAMA 1990;263:414-417.

20. Mintz PD, Nordine RB, Henry JB, Web WR: Expected hemotherapy in elective surgery. NY State J Med 1976;76:532-537.

21. Renner SW, Howanitz PJ, Bachner P: Preoperative autologous blood donation in 612 hospitals. Arch Pathol Lab Med 1992;116:613-619.

22. Goodnough LT, Riddell J, Kursh E, Resnick MI: Utilization and efficacy of autologous blood predeposit in radical prostatectomy with lymphapendectomy: Implications for blood conservation and physician education programs. Urology 1992;201-205.

23. Toy PTCY, Menozzi D, Strauss RG, Stehling LC, Kruskall M, AHN DK: Efficacy of preoperative donation of blood for autologous use in radical prostatectomy. Transfusion 1993;33:721-724.

24. Goodnough LT, Grishaber JE, Birkmeyer JD, Monk TG, Catalona WJ: Efficacy and cost-effectiveness of autologous blood predeposit in patients undergoing radical prostatectomy procedures. Blood (Abstract), Urology 1994; 44:226-231.

25. Goodnough LT, Vizmeg K, Verbrugge D: The impact of autologous blood ordering and blood procurement practices on allogeneic blood exposure in elective orthopaedic surgery patients. Am J Clin Path 1993, Urology 1994; 101:354-357.

26. Hull A, Wasman J, Goodnough LT: The effects of an autologous blood education program on physician transfusion behavior. Academic Medicine 1990;65:681.

27. Goodnough LT, Wasman J, Corlucci K, Chernoski A: Limitations to storing adequate autologous blood prior to elective surgery. Arch Surg 1989;124:494-496.

28. Goodnough LT: Blood conservation and blood transfusion practices: flip sides of the same coin. (Editorial) Ann Thor Surg, 1993;56:3-4.

29. Goodnough LT, Verbrugge D, Vizmeg K, Riddell J: Identifying elective orthopaedic surgical patients transfused with amounts of blood in excess of need: the transfusion-trigger" revisited. Transfusion 1992;32:648-653.

30. Goodnough LT, Vizmeg K, Robecks R, Schwarz A, Soegiarso W: Prevalence and classification of anemia in elective orthopaedic surgery patients: implications for blood conservation program. Vox Sang 1992;63:90-95.

31. McVay PA, Hoag MS, Lee SJ, Toy PTCY: Factors associated with successful autologous blood donation for elective surgery. Am J Clin Path 1992;97:304-308.

32. Goodnough LT, Rudnick S, Price TH, et al: Increased collection of autologous blood preoperatively with recombinant human erythropoietin therapy. N Engl J Med 1989;321:1163-1167.

33. Standards for Blood Banks and Transfusion Services. (15th edition) American Association of Blood Banks, Arlington VA, 1993:35.

34. Goodnough LT, Price TH, Rudnick S, Soegiarso RW: Preoperative red blood cell production in patients undergoing aggressive autologous blood phlebotomy with and without erythropoietin therapy. Transfusion 1992;32:441-445.

35. Price TH, Goodnough LT, Vogler W, et al: The impact of recombinant erythropoietin administration on the efficacy of autologous blood strategies in patients with low hematocrits. Blood (Abstract) 1992;80:219a.

36. Birkmeyer JD, Goodnough Lt, Aubuchon JP, Noordsij PG, Littenberg B: The cost-effectiveness of preoperative autologous blood donation for hip and knee replacement. Transfusion 1993;33:544-550.

37. Goodnough LT, Grishaber J, Monk T, Catalona WJ: Acute preoperative hemodilution in patients undergoing radical prostatecctomy: A case study analysis of efficacy. Transfusion (Abstract) 1993;33:60S

38. Goodnough LT, Saha P, Hirschler N, Yomtovian R: Autologous blood donation in non-orthopaedic surgery as a blood conservation strategy. Vox Sang 1992;63:96-101.

39. Goodnough LT, Bodner M, Martin S: Blood conservation and blood salvage. J Int Care Med 1994;9:86-92.

40. Goodnough LT: Evaluating the safety and efficacy of pharmacologic alternatives to blood. Ann Thor Surg 1993;56:1004-1005.

41. Goodnough LT, Price TH, Friedman KD, et al: A phase III trial of recombinant human erythropoietin therapy in non-anemic orthopaedic patients subjected to aggressive autologous blood phlebotomy: Dose, Response, Toxicity, and Efficacy. Transfusion 1994;34(1):66-71.

42. Goodnough LT, Price TH, Rudnick S: Iron-restricted erythropoiesis as a limitation to autologous blood donation in the erythropoietin-stimulated bone marrow. J Lab Clin Med 1991;188:289-295.

43. Goodnough LT, Vizmeg K, Riddell J, Soegiarso W: Prevalence of anemia in autologous blood donors prior to elective orthropaedic surgery: implictions for blood conservation programs. Vox Sang, 1992;63:96-101.

44. Brugnara C, Chambers LA, Malynn E, Goldberg MA, Kruskall MS: Red blood cell regeneration induced by subcutaneous recombinant erythropoietin: iron-deficient erythropoiesis in iron-replete subjects. Blood 1993;81:956-964.

45. Mercuriali F, Zanella A, Barosi G, et al: Use of erythropoietin to increase the volume of autologous blood donated by orthopaedic patients. Transfusion 1993;33:55-59.

46. Besarb A, Flaharty KK, Erslev AJ, et al: Clinical pharmacology and economics of recombinant erythropoietin in end-stage disease: The case for subcutaneous administration. J Am Soc Nephrol 1992;2(9):1405-16.

47. Hughes RT, Cotes PM, Oliver DO, et al: Correction of the anemia of chronic renal failure with erythropoietin: Pharmacokinetic studies in patients on haemodialysis and CAPD. Contrib Nephrol 1989;76:122-130.

48. Goodnough LT, Bravo J, Hsueh Y, Keating L, Brittenam GM: Red blood cell volume in autologous and homologous blood units: implications for risk/benefit assessment for autologous blood "crossover" and directed blood transfusion. Transfusion 1989;29:821-823.

49. Doolittle RF: Biotechnology - The enormous cost of success. N Engl J Med 1991;324:1360-1361.

50. Goodnough LT, Soegiarso RW, Birkmeyer JD, Welch HG: The economic impact of inappropriate blood transfusions in coronary artery bypass graft surgery. Am J Med 1993;94:1-5.

51. Birkmeyer JD, Aubuchon JP, Littenberg B, et al: The costs and benefits of preoperative autologous blood donation in elective coronary bypass surgery. Ann Thor Surg 1994; 57:161-169.

52. Eschbach JW, Egrie JC, Downing MR, Brown JK, Adamson JW: Correction of the anemia of end-stage renal disease with recombinatant human erythropoietin. N Engl J Med 1987;316:3-7.

53. Evans RW, Rader B, Manninen DL, Cooperative Multicenter EPO Clinical Trial Group: The quality of life of haemodialysis recipients treated with recombinant human erythropoietin. JAMA 1990;263:825-830.

54. Eschbach JB, Kelley MR, Haley NR, Abels RI, Adamson JW: Treatment of the anemia of progressive renal failure with recombinant human erythropoietin. N Engl J Med 1989;32:158-163.

55. Raine AEG: Hypertension, blood viscosity and cardiovascular morbidity in renal failure: ilmplications for erythropoietin therapy. Lancet 1988;1:97-100.

56. Harris WH, Sledge CB: Total hip and total knee replacement. N Engl J Med 1990;323:725-731.

57. Goodnough LT: Erythropoietin as a pharmacologic alternative to blood transfusion in the surgical patient. Trans Med Rev 1990;4:288-296.

58. Goodnough LT, Anderson KC, Kurtz S, et al: Indications and guidelines for the use of hematopoietic growth factors. Transfusion 1993;33(11):944-59.

59. Goodnough LT, Soegiarso RW, Geha AS: Blood lost and blood transfused in coronary artery bypass graft surgery: implications for blood conservation strategies. Surg Obstet Gyn 1993;177(4):345-51.

60. Goodnough LT, Vizmeg K, Marcus RE: Blood lost and blood transfused in elective orthopaedic surgery patients: Implications for blood conservation programs. Surg Obstet and Gyn 1993;176:235-238.

COMPONENT THERAPY

Keith F. O'Malley, M.D.

University of Medicine and Dentistry of New Jersey
Robert Wood Johnson Medical School at Camden
Cooper Hospital/University Medical Center
Camden, New Jersey

At a National Institutes of Health Consensus Conference in 1984, criteria for the transfusion of blood and components were developed and a policy of encouraging the appropriate use of component therapy, rather than whole blood, was adopted. This change was impelled by increasing concern over the risk of infectious disease transmission and the possibility of transfusioninduced immunosuppression,[1,2] as well as the recognition that it would be more economical and conserving of resources.

With few exceptions, the transfusion of fresh whole blood is no longer practiced, however current surgical practice has not always incorporated the latest recommendations or research findings regarding the appropriate use of blood components such as fresh frozen plasma (FFP), platelets, and cryoprecipitate. In fact, numerous studies have demonstrated that a significant number of blood and/or component transfusions are clearly unnecessary.[3,4] Part of the difficulty in reaching a consensus within the medical community on transfusion guidelines lies in the disparity between the internist's and the surgeon's viewpoint. Where the internist generally practices in a relatively controlled environment that allows time for reflection and carefully planned correction of abnormalities, the surgeon often must make decisions in situations where control, if not already lost, can be disrupted within seconds. There is a reluctance to wait for the results of directed laboratory studies to guide the need for component transfusion, since the delay incurred while obtaining these results is perceived as allowing the patient to further deplete the elements of the coagulation system. Often, therefore, the surgeon bases transfusion decisions on the more emotionally colored fears of what may happen. While this may be excusable in circumstances where blood loss is difficult to control and the rate of continuing losses is impossible to predict, it is feasible to develop and adhere to guidelines governing the use of blood products in the relatively well controlled elective setting. Certainly the routine use of *prophylactic* component transfusions needs to be reconsidered, if not, abolished. In those institutions where review of all component transfusions

Critical Issues in Surgery, Edited by A. C. Cernaianu et al.
Plenum Press, New York, 1995

131

are carried out and those physicians whose practices fell outside the accepted guidelines counselled, remarkable improvements in transfusion practice have been demonstrated. Such systems should be in place at each institution drawing on the region's blood supply.

BACKGROUND

Regional blood banks are charged with collecting, processing, and storing enough blood and blood products to meet the region's demand. The requirement that most processing take place within 46 hours of collection places considerable logistic strain on the regional center. This is compounded by the fact that each component has a limited shelf life. The regional center must therefore tightly coordinate collection and processing to ensure that adequate supplies of the various products are on hand.

Although it is feasible to estimate baseline needs fairly reliably, the peak demands that occur as a result of a medical or surgical emergency requiring the rapid provision of a large quantity of blood and components necessitates keeping some 30 to 50 percent more than baseline on hand. Maintaining this excess capacity is expensive and therefore each physician drawing on these resources should do so only when the products are clearly needed.

PLATELETS

Production requirements and demand for platelets largely dictate the pattern of whole blood collection in a regional blood service. The platelet rich plasma must be separated from the RBC concentrate within 4 hours of collection. The platelet packs are left with a residual plasma volume of 50 to 70 mL. Therefore administering a number of pooled platelet packs (generally 6 to 10) also results in supplying the patient with the equivalent of 1 or 2 units of fresh frozen plasma. Each unit contains at least 5.5×10^{10} platelets and will raise the patient's count by 5 to $8000/mm^3$. There are a few residual red blood cells present and, therefore, Rh compatibility must be checked prior to administering to women of childbearing age.

Aspirin interferes irreversibly with the platelet's ability to adhere to collagen, however the functional defect can be corrected by mixing with at least 20 percent normal platelets. Since platelets are usually administered in pools of 6 or more units, aspirin in generally only a problem in pediatric or single donor transfusions. Platelet function in donated blood is considerably better if at least 48 hours have elapsed since aspirin ingestion. Nonsteroidal antiinflammatory agents also interfere with platelet function, but this is reversible and only persists for some 6 to 8 hours.

The major demand for platelets result from thrombocytopenia caused by medical diseases such as ITP, TTP, secondary hypersplenism, etc., rather than surgical causes. It has been shown that a large percentage of platelets transfused surgery are unnecessary, even in a massive transfusion scenario.[5] Generally accepted guidelines[6,7] for the use of platelet transfusions in the surgical setting include:

1. Actively bleeding patients with thrombocytopenia or thrombocy-topathy if platelets are thought to be a contributing factor.
2. Documented thrombocytopenia after massive transfusion with clinically abnormal bleeding.
3. Possibly indicated to prepare certain patients (e.g. liver or renal insufficiency/failure) for invasive procedures, particularly if the central nervous system is involved.

There is no indication for prophylactic administration of platelets prior to open heart surgery. Their use is also not likely to be helpful if the platelet count is greater than $50,000/mm^3$ or the bleeding time is less than twice normal, unless there are other problems present.

Interestingly, resistance to changing practice guidelines is not restricted to the surgical community. Shulkin recently reported the experience of the hematology/oncology service at the University of Pennsylvania in attempting to lower the platelet transfusion trigger from $20,000/mm^3$ to $10,000/mm^3$. This change was well supported by the literature and was agreed upon by the entire group. However, the decision was reversed after two bleeding episodes during the first month under the revised guidelines, even though thrombocytopenia was not implicated as a causative factor.[8]

Depletion of platelets is the most common cause of nonsurgical bleeding in the setting of massive transfusion and is discussed in more detail in a succeeding section.

FRESH FROZEN PLASMA

The plasma portion should be separated from the cellular components within 68 hours of collection. After freezing, it may be kept at 18 degrees centigrade for up to a year. Depending on the time that it had been unfrozen, it may be relatively deficient in the labile factors V and VIII. If frozen promptly after separation, it will contain all the labile clotting factors, a normal potassium level, and few microaggregates when thawed. The presence of antiA and antiB isoagglutinins necessitates ABO compatibility matching prior to transfusion.

Braunstein and Oberman pointed out that it was difficult to establish acceptable guidelines for transfusion of FFP on the basis of the literature available in th early 1980's.[9] The NIH consensus conference found only limited indications for the use of FFP and specifically condemned the widespread (at that time) practice of using plasma as a volume expander or nutritional supplement. In surgical practice fresh frozen plasma should generally be used for replacement of multiple deficient factors (e.g. liver disease, massive transfusion, DIC) or when a specific deficiency has not yet been identified. Use should be reserved for those instances where there is active bleeding or the patient with a documented abnormal PT or PTT is facing an invasive procedure. It may also be used to rapidly correct the effects of warfarin.

Since thawing of FFP requires 20 to 30 minutes, it is necessary to anticipate the need for it while caring for the exsanguinating patient. In order to avoid unnecessarily thawing excess units during the "heat of battle", many centers have adopted massive transfusion protocols which call for the blood bank to automatically provide thawed FFP at regular intervals as the units of PRBC are administered.

CRYOPRECIPITATE

Cryoprecipitated Antihemophilic Factor is produced by collecting the precipitate formed when FFP is allowed to thaw at 4°C. It must be frozen within 6 hours of collection and can be stored at 18°C or below for a year. It is composed primarily of Factor VIII and fibrinogen, however the Factor VIII activity may vary widely. Other clotting factors are not contained in appreciable amounts. A platelet pack and cryoprecipitate can be prepared from a single unit of blood if there is at least 200 mL of cellfree plasma remaining after the platelets have been removed.

Each unit of cryoprecipitate contains 35 to 50 percent of the original Factor VIII and 20 to 25 percent of the plasma fibrinogen in about 5 percent of the original plasma volume. It must be administered through a filter due to the presence of insoluble debris composed of immunoglobulins, fibrino-protein, and coldinsoluble globulin. It also carries a hepatitis risk equal to that of a single unit of whole blood, and this is an additional argument against injudicious use.

Use of cryoprecipitate in surgery is extremely limited. Hypofibrino-genemia may develop during the course of massive transfusion if only FFP is administered. Many protocols therefore call for periodic transfusion of cryoprecipitate along with the more commonly employed blood components.

Beyond its use in directed replacement of Factor VIII or fibrinogen, cryoprecipitate is also used in preparation of *fibrin glue*, which is being investigated for its efficacy in a number of areas, such as repair of hepatic and splenic lacerations.[10]

MASSIVE TRANSFUSION

Massive blood loss or exsanguination is defined to be the *rapid* loss of at least one blood volume. Massive transfusion, on the other hand, is generally considered to be the *rapid* administration of 1.5 to 2 times the patient's blood volume. In massively transfused patients the main causes of coagulopathy are dilution of Factors V and VIII, dilutional thrombocy-topenia, and fibrinolysis.[11,12] Hypothermia developing during the course of a massive transfusion can cause profound disturbance of coagulation if the core temperature drops below 94°F and may actually be a more significant problem than the washing out of clotting factors.

During a massive transfusion, the platelet count rarely falls below 100,000/mm^3 if less than 20 units of packed red blood cells are given. Although there may be a transient drop, release of autologous platelets will usually maintain adequate levels . It has also been shown that there may be no need to give FFP unless more than 10 units of blood are given.[11] Therefore, it may be tempting to suggest that use of component therapy be guided by the results of laboratory studies, much as in the setting of elective surgery. Unfortunately it is difficult, if not impossible, to predict how easily the bleeding will be controlled. Since the onset of coagulopathy in the face of massive transfusion is associated with a high mortality, some system of presumptive component transfusion is used in many centers frequently dealing with such patients.

The goal of a massive transfusion protocol is twofold: to provide for provision of components as needed without requiring the preoccupied surgeon and anesthesiologist to expressly request them as PRBC are infused, as well as to minimize their excessive use.

The protocol is triggered at a certain point in the continuing administration of PRBC or at the insistence of the treating surgeon recognizing the presence of exsanguinating hemorrhage. From that point on the blood bank will continue to provide PRBC as requested, with components automatically sent along at some predetermined ratio.

A good model for component therapy has been devised by the University of Florida, Jacksonville.[11] After the protocol is triggered, the blood bank continues to send transfusion *packs* to the operating room, always staying one pack ahead of the demand. Each pack consists of five units of packed red blood cells, one unit of fresh frozen plasma, and five units of platelets. A protocol such as this has the virtue of minimizing the risk of falling behind in the replacement of clotting factors with resultant increase in ongoing blood loss.

This approach has been criticized by some as wasteful of blood bank resources while not necessarily beneficial to the patient. The University of Oregon, for example, uses laboratory studies to guide the administration of components and has reported exemplary results.[12] Clearly such a system represents the ultimate in management of massive transfusion, but demands an superlative effort from the blood bank and laboratory. Such an effort may be beyond the capacity of many institutions, leaving a *pack* system as the next best choice.

Interestingly, the status of the clotting system may not be the determining factor in the development of coagulopathy during massive transfusion. It is very difficult to maintain core body temperature in such situations, despite maintaining high operating room ambient temperature and warming of administered fluids. The deleterious effects of hypothermia and the ominous implications of its development are well known.[13,14] Reed et al[15] have shown that the kinetic activity of clotting cascade enzymes is critically dependant on temperature. If tests of clotting function are performed prior to warming the sample to normal temperature, the prolonged results may be taken to indicate a quantitative defect and lead to unnecessary component transfusion.

SUMMARY

The unnecessary administration of blood components has been well documented over the past decade. There are few indications for prophylactic administration of components and guidelines for their administration in everyday practice are well established. For the most part, the result of directed laboratory studies serves to establish the need for supplementation. This may be true even in the face of massive blood loss if the blood bank and laboratory services are sufficiently responsive.

REFERENCES

1. Rosemurgy AS, Hart MB, Murphy CG, et al: Infection after injury. Amer Surg 1992;58:104107.
2. Agarwal N, Murphy JG, Cayten CG, et al: Blood transfusion increases the risk of infection after trauma. Arch Surg 1993;128:171176
3. Goodnough LT, Soegiarso RW, Birkmeyer JD, et al: Economic impact of inappropriate blood transfusions in coronary artery bypass graft surgery. JAMA 1993; 94:509514.
4. Goodnough LT, Verbrugge D, Vizmeg K, et al: Identifying elective orthopedic patients transfused with blood volumes in excess of blood needs. Transfusion 1992;32:648653.
5. Reed RL, Ciavarella D, Heimbach DM, et al: Prophylactic platelet administration during massive transfusion. Ann Surg 1986;203:4048.
6. Practice parameters for the use of freshfrozen plasma, cryoprecipitate, and platelets. Development task force of the College of American Pathologists. JAMA 1994;271:777781.
7. Platelet Transfusion Therapy. NIH Consensus Conference. JAMA 1987; 257:17771780.
8. Shulkin DJ, Fox KR, Stadtmauer EA: Guidelines for prophylactic platelet transfusions: Need for a concurrent outcomes management system. Qual Rev Bull Dec 1992:477479.
9. Braunstein AH, Oberman HA: Transfusion of plasma components. Transfusion 1984;24:281286.
10. Murphy WG, Davies J, Eduardo A: The haemostatic response to surgery and trauma. Br J Aneaesth 1993;70:205213.
11. Frykberg ER, Dennis JW, Butcher JL: Massive transfusion. Trauma Quarterly 1993;10:1231.
12. Nelson CG, Otteson SP, Johnson RL: Massive transfusion. Lab Med 1991;22:9498.
13. Jurkovich GJ, Greiser WB, Luterman A, et al: Hypothermia in trauma victims: an ominous predictor of survival. J Trauma 1987;27:10191022.
14. Ferrara A, MacArthur JD, Wright HK, et al: Hypothermia and acidosis worsen coagulopathy in the patient requiring massive transfusion. Am J Surg 1990;160:515518.
15. Reed RL, Johnston TD, Hudson JD, et al: The disparity between hypothermic coagulopathy and clotting studies. J Trauma 1992;33:465470.

THE ANESTHESIOLOGIST'S VIEWPOINT: TRANSFUSION, HEMODILUTION AND COOPERATION

Linda Stehling, M.D.

Blood Systems, Inc.
Scottsdale, Arizona

It is estimated that two-thirds of red blood cell (RBC) transfusions are administered in the perioperative period.[1] One of the most significant changes in recent years is the increased use of autologous blood.[2,3] Blood for autologous transfusion may be donated preoperatively, recovered from the surgical wound intraoperatively and postoperatively, or withdrawn from the intravascular space into conventional blood bags when the patient is in the operating room. With the latter technique, termed acute normovolemic hemodilution (ANH), fluid is infused simultaneously to maintain normal intravascular volume. It is often appropriate to employ more than one autologous transfusion technique.

The surgeon determines whether blood is donated preoperatively and is responsible for blood recovery procedures, whereas the anesthesiologist performs hemodilution. Decisions regarding reinfusion of autologous blood are often made jointly. In the operating room, the anesthesiologist continuously monitors the patient's hemodynamic and intravascular volume status and oxygen delivery (DO_2) and usually determines when blood is transfused. However, the surgeon can best predict when hemostasis will be achieved. There is usually little disagreement about the indications for RBC administration when the surgeon and anesthesiologist function as a team. If they are not used to working together, controversy may arise. Legitimate differences of opinion also occur because the indications for transfusion are rarely absolute. Optimal patient management dictates that the surgeon and anesthesiologist discuss transfusion management prior to the occurrence of blood loss whenever possible.

Acute normovolemic hemodilution best exemplifies the need for cooperation between anesthesiologist and surgeon. The anesthesiologist should not unilaterally decide to employ ANH, particularly if the surgeon is unfamiliar with the technique. There are examples of surgeons being surprised to discover several units of the patient's blood neatly bagged and stored on the anesthesia cart! On the other hand, it is equally inappropriate

Critical Issues in Surgery, Edited by A. C. Cernaianu et al.
Plenum Press, New York, 1995

for a surgeon to ask the anesthesiologist to employ ANH in the absence of a thorough knowledge of the technique, adequate equipment, and assistance.

PRINCIPLES OF HEMODILUTION

Hemodilution entails the removal of blood immediately prior to or after induction of anesthesia and the simultaneous infusion of acellular fluid to maintain normal intravascular volume.[4] Crystalloid, colloid, or a combination of fluids can be infused. Colloid solutions are most often employed in Europe, whereas saline and Ringer's lactate are most often used in the United States. The amount of blood withdrawn depends upon the patient's blood volume, hematocrit (Hct) and overall physical condition. With limited hemodilution, the Hct is reduced to approximately 28 percent.[5] Extreme hemodilution refers to reduction of the Hct to less than 20 percent.[6]

The technique is used to decrease or eliminate the need for allogeneic (homologous) blood. Red blood cell loss is reduced when the Hct is lower. For example, the patient with a Hct of 45 percent who loses a liter of blood loses 450 mL of RBC. The RBC loss is 250 mL if the Hct is 25 percent. In addition, ANH is the only method of obtaining fresh whole autologous blood for transfusion.

Clinical Applications

Consideration should be given to employing ANH in surgical patients with adequate Hct who are expected to lose more than two units of blood. Children in whom blood loss is anticipated to exceed 20 percent of blood volume may also be appropriate candidates. Many cardiac surgeons employ ANH routinely, and the technique is becoming more popular for other types of surgery.

Appropriate patient selection is essential. Anemia is the major contraindication. It is generally inadvisable to employ ANH in patients with hemoglobin (Hb) values less than 11 g/dL. Patients with impaired renal function who cannot excrete large amounts of fluid are unsuitable candidates. Those with coronary artery disease or aortic stenosis having noncardiac surgery are usually excluded because the compensatory increase in cardiac output may not be possible or can be detrimental. When cardiopulmonary bypass is employed, pump flow can be altered to compensate for acute intravascular volume changes.[7] Limited monitoring capabilities and intravascular access contraindicate use of the technique.

Technical Aspects

Blood can be withdrawn from a central or large peripheral vein or an artery. The blood is collected in standard blood bags containing anticoagulant. When the blood is removed via a radial artery catheter, blood pressure can be transduced intermittently if a stopcock is incorporated in the system. Placement of a urinary catheter is essential because of the large fluid volumes infused and excreted. Urine output is also used as an indication of the adequacy of volume replacement.

The amount of blood (V) withdrawn is determined by the patient's estimated blood volume (EBV), initial Hct (Hct_o), the desired Hct following blood removal (Hct_f), and the average of the two (H_{av}):[8]

$$V = EBV \times \frac{Hct_o - Hct_f}{Hct_{av}}$$

For example, in a 70 kg patient with an EBV of 5L, Hct 45 percent, and lowest desired Hct of 27 percent, the volume of blood to be removed would be calculated as follows:

$$V = 5L \times \frac{45 - 27}{36} = 5L \times \frac{18}{36} = 2500 \text{ mL}$$

If crystalloid is used for replacement, the volume infused must be approximately three times the amount of blood removed because about two-thirds of the crystalloid moves into the extravascular space. Since colloids are retained within the intravascular space, the amount of albumin or other colloid administered is approximately equal to the volume of blood withdrawn. The primary advantage of using crystalloid, aside from cost, is that excess fluid can be excreted when a diuretic such as furosemide is administered before the blood is reinfused.

Each unit of blood must be labeled with the patient's name, hospital number, and the time it is withdrawn. The blood is usually kept in the operating room with the patient and maintained at room temperature to preserve platelet function. If it is anticipated that more than eight hours will elapse prior to reinfusion, it must be placed in an "igloo" with a coolant or in a monitored blood refrigerator. The blood is reinfused after major blood loss ceases, or sooner if necessary.

Estimations of blood loss and serial Hct determinations are used to guide transfusion. The minimally safe Hct depends on the patient's ability to compensate for decreased arterial oxygen content. Increased cardiac output is the primary compensatory mechanism and is due primarily to increased stroke volume. Heart rate does not usually increase in the absence of hypovolemia. Additional compensatory mechanisms are increased tissue oxygen extraction and diversion of blood flow to vital organs such as the heart and brain.[4]

SAFETY AND EFFICACY

The minimally safe Hct depends on the patient's ability to compensate for decreased arterial oxygen content. Hematocrits of approximately 20 percent are well tolerated by most patients as long as normovolemia is maintained.[9,10] Extreme hemodilution to average Hcts of 15 percent is safe in healthy adolescent patients.[6,11] However, there is little margin for error. Studies in animals with surgically-induced stenosis of the left anterior descending coronary artery have demonstrated marked myocardial dysfunction at mean Hb levels of 6 g/dL.[12] While the data should not be extrapolated to humans, they do offer some evidence that ANH may be contraindicated in patients with coronary artery disease having noncardiac surgery.

A decrease in allogeneic transfusion requirements of 20 to 90 percent has been reported for a variety of procedures, particularly when ANH is combined with other blood conservation techniques. One group reported that allogeneic transfusion was avoided in 60 to 90 percent of patients undergoing open heart surgery when blood conservation measures included ANH and reinfusion of shed mediastinal blood.[13] Other investigators have reported a less impressive, but significant, reduction in allogeneic transfusion when ANH, blood recovery, and reinfusion of mediastinal blood were employed.[7]

Four groups of investigators have reported favorable results when ANH was utilized during spinal surgery in children and adolescents. A reduction in allogeneic transfusion of 85 percent was shown in patients having Harrington instrumentation for scoliosis.[14] More recently, a similar decrease in allogeneic transfusion was reported when moderate ANH was employed during Cotrel-Dubousset instrumentation for scoliosis.[15] Extreme hemodilution to average Hcts of 15 percent reduced mean allogeneic transfusion requirements from approximately 4400 mL to 750 mL in another group of adolescents having Harrington instrumentation.[6] Intraoperative blood recovery was also employed in some patients. Unfortunately, historic controls were used in all of these studies. A significant decrease in the use of allogeneic blood components has been reported in patients having hepatic resection,[16] major colon surgery,[17] total hip arthroplasty,[18] and radical cystectomy.[19] In these studies, hemodiluted patients received one to three fewer units of allogeneic blood than control patients.

A recent prospective controlled comparison of ANH and preoperative autologous blood donation in a group of 50 patients having radical retropubic prostatectomy demonstrated equivalence of the two techniques in decreasing allogeneic transfusion requirements.[20] All patients had a standardized surgical procedure performed by the same surgeon and the anesthetic technique was standardized. The authors concluded that the results of the study could be applied to any elective procedure in which a blood loss of 1000 mL is anticipated.

Critics of ANH point out that the actual decrease in RBC loss may not be as great as predicted.[21] Considering errors inherent in the assumptions made regarding patients' blood volumes and the inaccuracy of blood loss estimations, it is surprising that the formula used to calculate the amount of blood to be withdrawn and the target Hct works so well.[8] Perhaps the most common explanation for little or no decrease in RBC loss and transfusion requirements is removal of an insufficient volume of blood. This may be compounded by reinfusing the blood prematurely. The greatest benefit is realized when three or more units are withdrawn and not transfused until the end of the surgical procedure. Even ardent proponents of ANH do not claim that it should be the first, and certainly not the only, blood conservation technique employed. There are, however, clinical circumstances when ANH is the best option.

Comparison with Other Autologous Transfusion Techniques

There is no doubt that ANH has several logistic advantages over other types of autologous transfusion. It is simpler and less expensive to obtain two to four units of blood by ANH than to have the patient donate a similar volume preoperatively. This is especially true for patients who live in rural areas without ready access to donor facilities and for those having surgery outside the communities in which they reside. Patients with cardiac, cerebrovascular, pulmonary and other systemic diseases may not be suitable candidates for predonation. However, withdrawal of blood in the operating room under carefully controlled conditions is a viable alternative for many of these "at risk" patients. When potential bacteremia associated with an indwelling urinary catheter or chronic osteomyelitis precludes predonation, ANH can be the ideal solution. If there is insufficient time for donation of an adequate number of units preoperatively, ANH can be employed as an additional blood conservation measure.

Hemodilution can be used as an adjunct to intraoperative and postoperative blood recovery, or as the sole technique when blood recovery is not feasible. Scheduling difficulties and personnel shortages may preclude use of blood recovery, particularly if cell processing apparatus is required. The presence of malignancy or infection may contraindicate the use of intraoperative blood recovery, but not ANH.

There are several reasons for underutilization of ANH, including the perception that it requires additional equipment, monitoring and personnel and prolongs the patient's time in the operating room. The monitoring required depends upon the degree of hemodilution and the physical condition of the patient. Placement of a pulmonary artery catheter is indicated for extreme ANH. Neither a pulmonary artery nor a central venous catheter is essential for moderate ANH. In the majority of cases where ANH is utilized, an arterial catheter would ordinarily be inserted for arterial pressure monitoring because of the hemodynamic changes and blood loss associated with the procedure.

Hemodilution may not be appropriate when the anesthesiologist is not part of an anesthesia care team because the usual scenario is for one person to anesthetize the patient and another to place the intravascular catheter and monitor blood withdrawal and fluid administration. An alternative is for a member of the surgical team to assist the anesthesiologist. Blood removal can usually be completed by the time the patient is anesthetized, the urinary catheter is placed, and the patient positioned and prepared for surgery.

Some physicians equate ANH with the acceptance of lower postoperative Hct values. Both contribute to decreasing allogeneic transfusion requirements. However, ANH implies the deliberate removal of blood from the intravascular space and its subsequent reinfusion, not merely the administration of intravenous fluid to maintain normovolemia at lower Hct levels. This distinction is important because low Hct levels that are safe in the operating room may not be tolerated in the postoperative period. Decreased oxygen consumption accompanies a properly conducted anesthetic, but oxygen requirements are often increased in the postoperative period. Shivering and sepsis are two of many factors that can increase oxygen consumption. While oxygenation is monitored and an increased inspired oxygen concentration is administered during surgery, this is not the case once the patient is discharged from the recovery room or intensive care unit.

SUMMARY

Hemodilution can reduce allogeneic transfusion requirements in some patients but it is not appropriate for all surgical patients. Proper patient selection and monitoring, removal of an adequate volume of blood, and cooperation between the surgeon and anesthesiologist are essential for the technique to be safe and effective.

REFERENCES

1. Office of Medical Applications of Research, National Institutes of Health. Perioperative red cell transfusion. JAMA 1988;260:2700.
2. Wallace EL, Surgenor DM, Hao HS, et al: Collection and transfusion of blood and blood components in the United States. Transfusion 1993;33;139.
3. Renner SW, Howanitz PJ, Bachner P: Preoperative autologous blood donation in 612 hospitals. Arch Pathol Lab Med 1992;116;613.
4. Stehling L, Zauder HL: Acute normovolemic hemodilution. Transfusion 1991;31:857.
5. Martin E, Hansen E, Peter K: Acute limited normovolemic hemodilution: A method for avoiding homologous transfusion. World J Surg 1987;11:52.
6. Martin E, Ott E: Extreme hemodilution in the Harrington procedure. Bibl Haematol 1981;47:322.
7. Scott WJ, Rode R, Castlemain B, et al: Efficacy, complications, and cost of a comprehensive blood conservation program for cardiac operation. J Thorac Cardiovasc Surg 1992;103:1001.
8. Gross JB: Estimating allowable blood loss: Correction for dilution. Anesthesiology 1973;58:277.
9. Jobes DR, Gallagher J: Acute normovolemic hemodilution. Int Anesthesiol Clin 1982;20:77.
10. Messmer K, Kreimeier U, Intaglietta M: Present state of intentional hemodilution. Eur Surg Res 1986;18:254.
11. Haberkern M, Dangel P: Normovolaemic haemodilution and intraoperative autotransfusion in children: experience with 30 cases of spinal fusion. Eur J Pediatr Surg 1991;1:30.
12. Spahn DR, Smith LR, Veronee CD, et al: Acute isovolemic hemodilution and blood transfusion. Effects on regional function and metabolism in myocardium with compromised coronary blood flow. J Thorac Cardiovasc Surg 1993;105:694.
13. Weniger J, Shanahn R: Reduction of blood bank requirements in cardiac surgery. J Thorac Cardiovasc Surg 1982;82:142.
14. Kafer ER, Isley MR, Hansen T, et al: Automatic acute normovolemic hemodilution reduces blood transfusion for spinal fusion. Anesth Analg 1986;65:S86.
15. Olsfanger D, Jedeikin R, Metser U, et al: Acute normovolaemic haemodilution and idiopathic scoliosis surgery: effects on homologous blood requirements. Anaesth Intens Care 1993;21:429.
16. Sejourne P, Poirier A, Meakins JL, et al: Effect of hemodilution on transfusion requirements in liver resection. Lancet 1989;2:1380.
17. Rose D, Coutosftides T: Intraoperative normovolemic hemodilution. J Surg Res 1981;31:375.
18. Roseberg B, Wulff K: Regional lung function following hip arthroplasty and preoperative normovolemic hemodilution. Acta Anaesth Scand 1979;23:242.
19. Atallah MM, Abdelbaky SM, Saied MM: Does timing of hemodilution influence the stress response and overall outcome? Anesth Analg 1993;76:113.

20. Ness PM, Bourke DL, Walsh PC: A randomized trial of perioperative hemodilution versus transfusion of preoperatively deposited autologous blood in elective surgery. Transfusion 1992;32:226.

21. Brecher M, Rosenfeld M: Computer modeling of acute normovolemic hemodilution (ANH). Transfusion 1993;33:S234.

ENDOVASCULAR SURGERY

Sushil K. Gupta, M.D., Nissage Cadet, M.D., and
Thomas K. Whang, M.D.

Metro West Medical Center
Farmingham, Massachusetts

INTRODUCTION

The quest to recanalize occluded peripheral arteries began in the 19th and early 20th century and benefitted significantly from the discovery of anticoagulation drugs such as heparin and dicumarol. The first successful disobliteration by thromboendarterectomy was reported by Dos Santos in 1946[1] and later popularized by Wylie[2] and others in the 1950s. The field of vascular surgery experienced accelerated growth with thrombo-endarterectomy and reconstructive arterial bypasses.

Endovascular surgery began in the early 1960s when Dotter and Judkins[3] reported the first attempts at dilating arterial occlusive lesions and grew with the development of balloon catheters by Gruntzig.[4] Although fraught with problems originally, percutaneous transluminal angioplasty (PTA) has now become a major tool in the management of vascular disease. The ability to intervene percutaneously in the treatment of peripheral arterial disease in areas remote from the entrance site may offer many advantages as an alternative or adjunct to surgical procedures.

Endovascular surgery may be defined as a therapeutic discipline that uses a single point of entry into the vascular tree to transport devices for intraluminal imaging and intervention remote from the site of entry. This entry may be percutaneous or by limited surgical exposure. The main purpose of endovascular surgery is to open or widen stenotic or occluded channels in the vascular tree directly or to aid the performance of other vascular procedures. More recently, intraluminal stents and grafts have been used to treat aneurysmal disease and to bridge gaps in the occluded arterial tree.

BALLOON ANGIOPLASTY

Percutaneous transluminal angioplasty (PTA) is the most popular and accepted means of angioplasty. The concept and technique of PTA are well

Critical Issues in Surgery, Edited by A. C. Cernaianu et al.
Plenum Press, New York, 1995

described in many textbooks. It is essentially similar to Gruntzigs original technique in the 1974 report. PTA is now an accepted modality in the treatment of atherosclerotic vascular disease. It is widely used for the dilatation of vascular stenosis or recanalization of occluded arteries. Numerous reports in the surgical and radiological literature attest to the clinical success and utility of this procedure. Tunis et al.[5] reported an increase of more than 24 fold in PTA from 1979 to 1989 in the state of Maryland. Advances in the technology of catheters, guidewires and advances in technique have all improved the overall safety and efficacy of the procedure.

In spite of this success, the mechanism of PTA is still unknown. The most accepted explanation is that balloon angioplasty creates a disruption, splitting and a separation of atheroma from the media of the artery. PTA creates a controlled injury by fracturing the plaque, thus causing damage to the endothelial layer. As the skills and experience of clinicians (vascular surgeons and radiologists) improve, the indications for PTA have been liberalized. Currently, the most common indications for PTA are claudication, rest pain, tissue loss and limb salvage, and as an adjunct to reconstructive vascular surgery. Some of the indications are relative, controversial and debatable. PTA may be applied to any vessel given the technical feasibility with regard to size or lumen of the vessel. Nonetheless, the technical and clinical results of PTA are site dependent. For example, the results of balloon angioplasty for iliac artery stenosis are different than those for femoropopliteal disease.

Two criteria are used to define the results for PTA: 1) improvement of symptoms and 2) documented measurable findings. A clinical success is achieved if there is symptomatic improvement by at least one level such as asymptomatic, mild claudication, incapacitating claudication and rest pain. A measurable laboratory improvement such as an increase in ankle brachial index (ABI) of 0.10, change of the pulse volume recording (PVR) wave form from monophasic to biphasic and to triphasic. The clinical evaluation differs from the technical evaluation. A technical success is determined angiographically by improvement of the luminal diameter by 20 percent.

LASER ANGIOPLASTY

PTA has technical limitations as the procedure may fail to remove or destroy the atherosclerotic plaque. The segment of artery involved can restenose or reocclude. In addition, the endothelial damage created by the cracking of the plaque may be the focal point for rethrombosis. Laser has had good success as a modality in surgical applications, especially ophthalmologic procedures. For many years, laser was seen as a major advancement and has been investigated for potential applications in the treatment of vascular diseases.

To use laser appropriately and effectively, it is necessary to understand the principle. It is not the scope of this chapter to explain the principles of laser, but suffice it to say that laser is a light source whose photons are emitted parallel to and in phase with each other. Therefore, intensity is not decreased and pinpoint accuracy is obtained. Laser energy can be produced by many different devices. Argon, CO_2, and YAG lasers are the most commonly used. As a light source, laser emits energy in the form of heat. The objective of laser therapy is the precise control of thermal heat. Tissue ablation occurs because of the process of absorption which is key to effective laser use. Tissue ablation through the intraluminal application of laser energy may indeed provide a minimal intervention to recanalize occluded arteries. The goal of laser in the treatment of vascular disease is to accomplish atheroma ablation without damaging surrounding normal artery.

ATHERECTOMY

PTA though successful for short stenotic lesions, is not as effective for long stenoses or occlusions. Following balloon angioplasty, the intraluminal surface is left rough with fractures in the plaque. In addition, the fact that plaque material is not removed, may contribute to the high recurrence rates following balloon angioplasty. To improve the overall results, emphasis has been placed on finding a new device to remove plaque material by either laser or mechanical means, particularly the atheromatous plaque. The initial success achieved with several atherectomy devices have engendered great enthusiasm in their application as a tool in the endovascular surgical armamentarium. However, their role in the management of atherosclerotic disease is not yet defined and remains to be determined by further refinements, technical advances and clinical experience. There are several atherectomy devices actually available on the market. Each offers its own unique features with advantages and disadvantages. The complication rate for atherectomy procedures range from 15 to 30 percent.[6] The most important complications are perforation, embolization, thrombosis, restenosis and hemogloburia. As with any technologic modality, limitations have been outlined in the area of long stenotic lesions and tortuous small vessels have a high incidence of restenosis and failure.

Preliminary reports of the Simpson and directional atherectomy catheters, the Auth rotoblater and transluminal extraction catheter (TEC) (Inventional Technologies, Inc., San Diego, CA) have been good, but most studies thus far have been experimental and at best, short-term. Further long-term clinical and comparative studies are necessary.

Auth Rotary Atherectomy Device

The Auth Rotary Atherectomy device (Heart Technology, Inc., Bellevue, WA) is one of the devices available using a diamond studded burr. The device employs the principle of differential cutting that allows the burr to cut only into the hard plaque rather than the normal elastic wall. The particles generated by the device are not removed, but are allowed to remain in the circulation to be eliminated by the reticulo-endothelial system. The size of the particles is determined by the size of the diamond chips in the burr and has been shown to be less than 8 m in 97 percent of cases. These particles pass harmlessly through the circulatory system.

In canine and cadaver experiments, the resulting arterial lumen was smooth and polished with smooth endpoints. Based on these satisfactory results in human cadaver arteries, three medical centers entered into

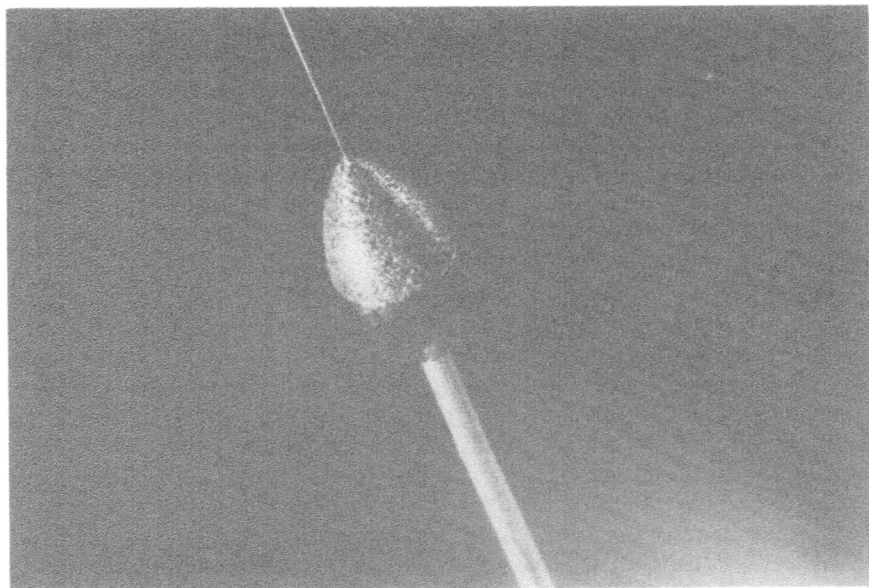

Figure 1. Close-up view of the Rotablator Tip exposes the microscopic Diamond Crystals which polish the inner surface of the bodys arteries while gently ablating atherosclerotic plaque. A tiny hole permits passage of an independent guidewire.

clinical trials. The present report deals with our experience with early and intermediate results with the atherectomy of infrainguinal arteries using the Auth Rotator. This is a multicenter trial for the University of California at Los Angeles, Montefiore Medical Center and Stanford University. The results were published in the *Journal of Vascular Surgery* in 1994.[6]

During the period from August 1987 to December 1990, selected patients presenting with infrainguinal atherosclerosis who were candidates for femoropopliteal or distal bypasses were offered an alternate treatment using the Auth atherectomy device. Seventy-nine atherectomy procedures were performed on 107 stenotic or occluded arterial segments on 79 limbs of 72 patients. Thirty four patients (43 percent) were treated for significant claudication as the only symptom, 44 (56 percent) presented with rest pain or non-healing ulcers, and one patient had an asymptomatic failing graft (1 percent). These lesions were classified by the length of the lesion, i.e., less than or greater than 10 cm. Seventy arterial segments were less than 10 cm in length and 37 were longer than 10 cm. The mean age was 69 years. There were 53 male and 26 female patients. These patients were typical peripheral vascular disease patients with a high incidence of risk factors including hypertension (76 percent), coronary artery disease (63 percent), diabetes (46 percent), smoking (57 percent), and previous vascular surgery (56 percent). The device is pictured in Figure 1.

Figure 2 shows the burr in place in the arterial lumen adjacent to the plaque. A small console is used to control and monitor the burr RPM. There is also a disposable burr advancer unit.

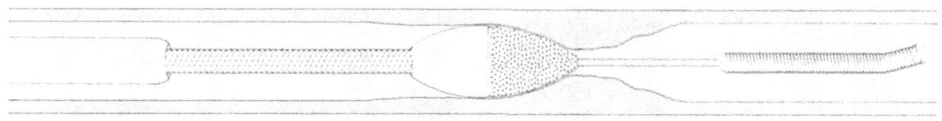

Figure 2. Rotablator device

All procedures were performed in the operating room with a vascular surgeon and a radiologist working as a team. An arteriotomy at the chosen site was made by the vascular surgeon. Under fluoroscopic control the radiologist places a suitable sized sheath for passage of the guidewire and the burr. Most lesions are easily traversed by a normal guide wire. Occasionally, a glide guide wire is used to pass difficult or occluded lesions. This guide wire is exchanged for a stiffer guidewire supplied with a device which acts as a rail to place the burr in proximity with the lesion. The speed of the burr is maintained by an air driven turbine controlled by the console.

Intravenous dextran mixed with paperavine was administered postoperatively for 24 to 48 hours in the first 12 cases of the group from University of California, Los Angeles. However, full heparinization was employed in all subsequent cases. All patients were started on aspirin preoperatively which is continued indefinitely.

Postoperative evaluation was analyzed with regard to intraoperative, in-hospital and late success. Intraoperative angiographic success was defined as a decrease of the stenotic lesion to less than 25 percent of the normal luminal diameter. In-hospital success related to clinical improvement in claudication with resolution of symptoms and a increase in ABI by at least 0.15. Late success related to the maintenance of the criteria of clinical success. Intraoperative angiographic success was quite excellent and is shown in Table 1.

There were nine initial technical failures and an additional nine in-hospital thromboses to give an initial clinical success rate of 77 percent. There were no deaths in this population. There were 26 complications within

Table 1. Angiographic Success

Lesion site	No. of lesions	No. of successful procedures	%
Iliac (>10 cm)	2	1	50
Superficial femoral	45	38	84
≤10 cm	24	21	88
>10 cm	21	17	81
Popliteal	29	25	82
≤10 cm	15	13	87
>10 cm	14	12	86
Tibial/peroneal (≤10 cm)	31	19	61
Total Lesions	07	82	77
Total No. of limbs/patients	70/79		89

30 days with ten amputations in total. Two limb losses among the ten amputees were device related. The other complications included four cases of hematoma of the arteriotomy site, one pseudoaneurysm and one wound infection. Transient hemoglobinuria occurred in ten patients however it did not cause renal failure in any patient. Eight cases of microemboli were observed. Three were considered significant and four presented as maculopapular rash. In two patients cutaneous necrosis occurred; in one of these, toe gangrene necessitated toe amputation. These embolic complications occurred in either patients with long lesions or when a large burr size was used. This problem was obviated in the last five cases by passing the burr retrograde through the distal popliteal artery and then discarding the first 50 cc of blood collected through the sheath before restoring circulation.

The secondary life table was achieved by re-atherectomy or balloon angioplasty for restenosis but did not improve substantially. When we compared the life table patency of claudicants with those of limb salvage patients, there was no significant difference. When we compared the patients based on the length of the lesion, the life table patency with shorter lesions was better, but not significantly. Based on this experience, we concluded that 1) the role of Auth rotoblator in treating peripheral arteries is not proven; 2) if this device is to have any role in treating short lesions, this role should be decided based on randomized comparisons with balloon angioplasty; 3) we have seen that clinically significant emboli can occur, but most of these can be avoided by the retrograde passage of the burr.

ANGIOSCOPY

Many studies have clearly demonstrated that the routine use of angioscopy as a monitoring procedure in infrainguinal bypass procedures in clinically useful, safe and effective. Its use is of great value for valve ablation in *in-situ* vein bypass. The blind approach of valvulotomy for *in-situ* and nonreversed vein conduits is associated with a significant number of infrainguinal graft failure. Thickened or sclerotic valves, residual valves, intraluminal webs, bands and strands are the most commonly observed findings. Angioscopically assisted interventions of these defects allowed improvement of the quality of the vein graft. Furthermore, angioscopy can be invaluable in completion evaluation of distal anastomoses especially in the inframaelleolar position. Intraoperative angiography has many limitations in evaluating small vessels.

REFERENCES

1. Dos Santos JC: Sur la desobstruction des thomboses arterielles anciennes. Mem Acad Chir 1946;147(73):409.
2. Wylie EJ: Thromboendarterectomy for arteriosclerotic thrombosis of major arteries. Surgery 1952;32:275.
3. Dotter CT, Judkins MP: Transluminal recanalization in occlusive disease of the leg arteries. GP 1968;1:98-106.
4. Gruntzig A, Hopff H: Perkutane Rekanalisation chronischer arterieller Verschlussse mit einem neuen Dilationskatheter: Modification der Dott-Technik. Dtsch Med Wochenscher 1974;99:2502-2505.

5. Tunis SR, Bass EB, Steinberg EP: The use of angioplasty, bypass surgery, and amputation in the management of peripheral vascular disease. New Eng J Med 1991;325:556-562.
6. Collaborative Rotablator Atherectomy Group. Peripheral atherectomy with the rotablator: a multicenter report. J Vasc Surg 1994;19:509-515.

HYPOMAGNESEMIA AS A PREDICTOR OF MORTALITY IN CRITICALLY ILL TRAUMA PATIENTS

Philip C. Wry, M.D., Anthony J. Mure, M.D., and
Steven E. Ross, M.D.

University of Medicine and Dentistry of New Jersey
Robert Wood Johnson Medical School
Cooper Hospital/University Medical Center
Camden, New Jersey

Hypomagnesemia has been described as *one of the most common electrolyte abnormalities of hospitalized patients* as well as *the most under diagnosed electrolyte deficiency in current medical practice.*[1,2] Low serum magnesium concentration has been shown to be a common finding in medical, postoperative, and pediatric ICU patients, and to be associated with higher mortality and poorer outcome in these patients. Rubiez et al have shown a 63% incidence of hypomagnesemia detected on admission of 400 acutely ill medical patients being associated with increased mortality.[3] Chernow et al reported hypomagnesemia in 61% of 193 postoperative ICU patients, having a higher mortality than similarly ill normo-magnesemic patients, with severe hypomagnesemia (<1 mEq/L) being clinically important.[4] Ryzen et al studied 94 medical ICU admissions, finding a 65% incidence of magnesium deficiency in patients with normal creatinine.[5] Broner et al demonstrated a significantly poorer outcome, as measured by either survival or ICU length of stay, in 98 critically ill pediatric patients with either hypermagnesemia (43.3%) or hypocalcemia (17%).[6]

We hypothesized that hypomagnesemia would be associated with increased mortality in critically injured patients. The objectives of this study were to determine the incidence of hypomagnesemia on admission to a Trauma ICU, to elucidate its clinical importance and to determine its impact on outcome, in relation to other variables.

The records of 178 patients admitted to a Trauma ICU at a level 1 Trauma Center were retrospectively analyzed. Magnesium levels were drawn on admission to the ICU after resuscitation evaluation and initial treatment was performed in the receiving area or operating room. No magnesium or calcium was given therapeutically prior to drawing the first

Critical Issues in Surgery, Edited by A. C. Cernaianu et al.
Plenum Press, New York, 1995

Table 1. Patterns of Injury

Type of major injury*	No. of Patients (%)
Head	63 (35%)
Chest	9 (5%)
Abdominal	24 (13%)
Orthopedic	37 (21%)
Facial	2 (1%)

*Major defined as AIS≥3; BP = Blood pressure; ETOH = ethanol

magnesium levels (except calcium from lactated Ringers solution.) Nutritional therapy was not instituted prior to drawing initial magnesium levels.

Hypomagnesemia was defined as less than 1.8 mEq/L. Laboratory measurements were performed using the calmagnite reagent with the Boehringer Mannheim/Hitachi 747 chromophore absorbance analyzer. The normal range for serum magnesium was reported as 1.8 to 2.4 mEq/L. Hemolysis falsely elevates results, due to elution of magnesium from red cells, and is reported by the laboratory.

Student's t-test and contingency table analysis (chi square or Fischer's exact) were used for statistical analysis.

The majority of patients sustained blunt trauma (89%); most of these patients were motor vehicle occupants (61%). The pattern of injury is what would be expected in a blunt trauma population, with predominantly major head, chest, and orthopedic injuries[7] (Table 1). Seventy-two percent of penetrating injuries (10% of total cases) were gunshot wounds (Table 2).

The mean injury severity score (ISS) was 17 ± 13, the mean revised trauma score (TS) was 9 ± 3, the mean Glasgow coma scale was 10 ± 5 (Table 3). These results indicate moderate physiologic and neurologic derangements associated with severe anatomic injury.

The mean magnesium level was 1.5 mEq/L with a range of 0.6 to 4.0 mEq/L. Admission hypomagnesemia was found in 76% (136/178) of pa-

Table 2. Mechanisms of Injury

Blunt		158
	MVA Occupant	96
	Pedestrian	18
	Bicyclist	2
	Motorcyclist	8
	Assault	6
	Fall	21
	Other	7
Penetrating		18
	GSW	13
	SW	3
Other		2
	Drowning	1
	Burn	1

MVA = Motor vehicle accident; GSW = Gun shot wound; SW = Stab wound.

Table 3. Severity Indicators in Study Population

Mean ISS	17 ± 13
Mean TS	9 ± 3
Mean GCS	10 ± 5
Mean ICU Admission Systolic BP	126 ± 27

ISS = Injury severity score; TS = Trauma scene; GCS = Glasgow coma score; BP =Blood pressure. Data presented as mean ± standard deviation.

tients. Normal magnesemia levels were found in 22% (40/138) of patients. Overall mortality was 12% (22/178). Magnesium deficiency was observed in 82% (18/22) of the mortalities. Severe hypomagnesemia (<1.0 mEq/L) was found in 6 patients; there were no mortalities in this subgroup.

Hypermagnesemia (>2.4 mEq/L) was found in only 2 patients, one of these patients died. The highest magnesium of our group was 4.0 mEq/L found in a drowning victim who was a non-survivor.

There was no statistically significant correlation between hypomagnesemia and mortality, as well as no statistical significance in the mean magnesium levels of survivors and non-survivors.

In comparing the hypomagnesemic and normomagnesemic groups, there was no statistical significance in relation to the ISS, revised TS, Glasgow coma scale, resuscitation fluid or blood transfusions, blood pressure on admission to and discharge from trauma admitting area, acute ethanol intoxication (ETOH>100 mg/dL), hemoglobin, and serum levels of sodium, potassium or phosphorus. There was a statistically significant difference in the non-ionized calcium levels between the two groups. These values were not corrected for albumin, and are of uncertain clinical significance. Although ethanol is known to cause hypomagnesemia, there was no statistically significant difference in hypomagnesemia between intoxicated and nonintoxicated patients.

Magnesium is the second most common intracellular cation, and the fourth most common cation in the body. Magnesium is a metabolic co-factor in over 300 enzymatic reactions, including nucleic acid, protein synthesis, and energy utilization. It is required in cellular phosphate transfer reactions (sodium-potassium adenosine-triphosphate pump, calcium-ATPase pump, proton pump). Magnesium participates in cellular second messenger systems and regulation of vascular smooth muscle tone.[8]

Only 1.3% of magnesium is in the extracellular fluid, 31% is intracellular and 67% is in bone. Approximately 1/3 of magnesium from bone is available for exchange with the extracellular fluid. Fifty-five percent of plasma magnesium is free (ionized). The remainder is bound to albumin, globulins, and chelated to salts. Currently, measurement of ionized magnesium is not readily available for use in clinical practice. Therefore, circulating magnesium may not adequately reflect physiologically active (free or ionized) or cellular stores of magnesium. Other approaches to diagnosing magnesium levels are: 1) the serum ultrafilterable (protein-free); 2) mononuclear cell (lymphocytes and erythrocytes) magnesium levels;[8,9] 3) ionized magnesium in whole blood, serum, and plasma;[10] and 4) intracellular ionized magnesium.[11]

Hypomagnesemia may be caused by: 1) decreased intake, 2) increased losses both gastrointestinal and renal, 3) drug-induced, and 4) alterations in distribution.[9] Distribution changes are probably the cause in the acute trauma setting.

Clinical signs of hypomagnesemia are protean manifesting primarily as cardiovascular and neurologic derangements. Cardiovascular manifestations involve the entire gamut of tachyarrhythmias ranging from premature ventricular contractions to ventricular fibrillation, including sudden cardiac death. There is a clinically significant association with myocardial ischemia, infarction and spasm, as well as a host of other cardiac disorders. The multiple associated EKG changes are similar to those seen with potassium deficiency.[8,13]

Neuromuscular and neurological derangements of magnesium deficiency present primarily as excitability ranging from hyperreflexia to tetany and seizures. Respiratory skeletal and smooth muscle weakness may lead to prolonged ventilator dependance. Neurobehavioral symptoms vary from confusion to frank psychosis. Anemia and impaired renal and parathyroid function are also associated with hypomagnesemia. Neonates are particularly sensitive to magnesium deficiency.[8,13]

In light of all the clinical symptomatology associated with hypomagnesemia and because magnesium is involved in so many important cellular processes, it is not surprising that magnesium deficiency can have serious and fatal consequences.

It is evident that trauma patients are vigorously resuscitated in the admitting area, throughout their work-up and in the operating room prior to arrival in the intensive care unit. Fluid resuscitation and blood transfusions could account for a percentage of our hypomagnesemic ICU admissions, secondary to distributive changes, but no statistically significant difference in blood or other resuscitation fluids was shown between the normomagnesemic groups. This has led to an interest in investigating magnesium levels in the trauma admitting area as part of a prospective outcome study.

Although ethanol is known to cause hypomagnesemia[8], there was no statistically significant difference in hypomagnesemia between intoxicated and non intoxicated patients (ETOH>100mg/dL).

There has been little research regarding adequate therapy for hypomagnesemia, despite the high prevalence of magnesium deficiency in the ICU and the importance of its associated morbidity and mortality. Current research indicates that serum magnesium may be normal in the presence of significant intracellular deficiency. Futhermore, total body magnesium repletion may not be achieved through the correction of subnormal serum magnesium concentration to normal values.[14] This raises extremely important questions about magnesium supplementation in critically ill patients.

Our study has shown a slightly higher percentage of critically ill trauma patients having hypomagnesemia than acutely and critically ill medical, post-operative, and pediatric patients. However, our study did not demonstrate a clinically significant association of magnesium disorders to mortality and poor outcome, as reported in previous studies reviewed. This may be related to the acute nature of the disease process, rather than the chronic disorders seen in the medical ICU setting. Prospective studies, including studies of tissue, intracellular, and ionized magnesium levels are necessary to determine the importance of hypomagnesemia in critically injured patients as well as other critically ill patient populations.

REFERENCES

1. Whang R. Magnesium deficiency: Pathogenesis, prevalence and clinical implications. Am J Med 1987;82(S3A):24-29.
2. Wacker WEC. Measurement of magnesium in human tissues and fluids: A historical perspective. Magnesium 1987;6:61-64.
3. Rubeiz GJ, Thill-Baharozian M, Hardie D, et al. Association of hypomagnesemia and mortality in acutely ill medical patients. Crit Care Med 1993;21:203-209.
4. Chernow B, Bamberger S, Stoiko M, et al. Clinical hypomagnesemia in patients in post-operative intensive care. Chest 1989;95:391-397.
5. Ryzen E, Wagers PW, Singer FR, et al. Magnesium deficiency in a medical ICU population. Crit Care Med 1985;13:19-21.
6. Broner CW, Sti Dham Gl, Westenkirchner DF, et al. Hypermagnesemia and hypocalcemia as predictors of high mortality in critical ill pediatric patients. Crit Care Med 1990;18:921-928.
7. Moore EE, Mattox KL, Feliciano DV. Patterns of injury. In: Wounds and Injuries. Moore E, Mattox KL, Feliciano DV (eds) Appleton & Lange, Norwalk, Conn., 1991, pp 81-93.
8. Salem M, Munoz R, Chernow B. Hypomagnesemia in critical illness, a common and clinically important problem. Critical Care Clinics 1991;7:225-252.
9. Chernow B, Smith J, Rainey T, et al. Hypomagnesemia: implications for the critical care specialist. Crit Care Med 1982;10:193-196.
10. Altura BT, Shirey TL, Young CC. A new method for the rapid determination of ionized magnesium in whole blood, serum and plasma. Meth Find Exp Clin Pharmacol 1992;14(4):297-304.
11. Murphy E. Measurement of intracellular ionized magnesium. Miner Electrolyte Metab 1993;19:250-258.
12. Alvarez-Leefmans FJ, Giraldez F, Gamino SM: Intracellular free magnesium in excitable cells: Its measurement and its biologic significance. Can J Phisiol Pharmacol 1987;65:915-925.
13. Schwartz GR. Endocrine and metabolic emergencies. In: Principles and practice of emergency medicine. Schwartz GR, Clayten CG, et al. (eds), Lea & Febiger, Philadelphia, Pa., 1992, pp 2076-2079.
14. Olerich M, Rude R. Should we supplement magnesium in critically ill patients? New Horizons 1994;2:186-192.

ABDOMINAL PARACENTESIS

Alan D. Miranda, M.D. and David R. Gerber, D.O.

University of Medicine and Dentistry of New Jersey
Robert Wood Johnson Medical School
Cooper Hospital/University Medical Center,
Camden, New Jersey

Abdominal paracentesis is a procedure for percutaneously removing abdominal fluid for diagnostic and/or therapeutic purposes. At the present time paracentesis is primarily utilized in the evaluation of a variety of intra-abdominal pathologies as well as for therapeutic purposes. In the past this procedure was utilized in the evaluation of abdominal trauma (four-quadrant tap), but it has since been replaced by the technique of peritoneal lavage.

Paracentesis is indicated in any patient with new onset ascites. Some authors advocate paracentesis in all patients with known ascites each time they are admitted to the hospital.[1,2] The development of new clinical or laboratory evidence of infection should prompt the performance of this procedure, even if it has been performed previously. Signs or symptoms suggesting infection are variable and include fever, leukocytosis, hypotension, abdominal pain, renal failure or encephalopathy. In 10 to 27% of cases, infected ascitic fluid is asymptomatic.[1]

Therapeutic indications for paracentesis include relief of discomfort and relief of respiratory embarrassment from impaired diaphragmatic movement.

CONTRAINDICATIONS

In the past coagulopathy has been considered a contraindication to paracentesis. This is no longer felt to be true, and currently, overt disseminated intravascular coagulopathy (DIC) or fibrinolysis should be the only hematologic criteria for excluding paracentesis. Consistent with this position, the practice of giving fresh frozen plasma (FFP) for low grade coagulopathy before the procedure is not supported by available data.[1,2] Other contraindications to performing paracentesis include infection of the abdominal wall in the area of proposed puncture, severe gaseous distension or bowel obstruction and poor patient cooperation. A surgical scar in the

Critical Issues in Surgery, Edited by A. C. Cernaianu et al.
Plenum Press, New York, 1995

159

area of proposed paracentesis requires selection of a different site since bowel may be adherent to the scar.

DIFFERENTIAL DIAGNOSIS

The differential diagnosis of the etiology of ascites includes parenchymal liver disease, infection, malignancy, congestive heart failure, tuberculosis, pancreatitis, connective tissue disease and nephrotic syndrome.

DIAGNOSTIC TESTS

Routine tests performed on ascitic fluid obtained should include cell count, albumin and culture. Gram staining of ascites, as well as determination of total protein, amylase, LDH, and glucose are often indicated in specific situations. Tests which are sometimes requested but generally considered unhelpful are pH, lactate, cholesterol, and fibronectin. Cytology and tuberculosis smears should be done only in the appropriate clinical setting (e.g., when evaluating a patient with a known underlying disease or when malignancy or tuberculosis are truly part of the differential diagnosis).

Appearance of Fluid

Ascitic fluid is ordinarily slightly yellow in color and transparent. Particulate matter tends to increase the cloudiness of the fluid. Neutrophils are the most common cause of cloudy or turbid ascites. Ascites with an absolute white blood cell (WBC) count of less than 1000/mL are nearly clear, counts over 5000/mL usually result in cloudy fluid, and ascites with counts greater than 50,000/mL appears purulent.[2] Ascites which has a bloody appearance usually demonstrates red blood cell (RBC) counts greater than 20,000/mL. Trauma during the paracentesis is the usual etiology of bloody ascites. A traumatic tap is indicated by blood that clots or is heterogeneous in the ascitic fluid. Blood that is homogeneous or does not clot indicates non-traumatic ascites or ascites due to remote trauma.[2] Potential etiologies of non-traumatic, bloody ascites include portal hypertension, hepatocellular carcinoma, peritoneal carcinomatosis and tuberculosis.[2]

WBC Count

A WBC count greater than 500/mL or a polymorphonuclear cell (PMN) count greater than 250/mL are generally considered the upper limits of normal. Counts above these levels are evidence for peritoneal inflammation.[9,11] False elevation of the WBC count can occur by two primary mechanisms. A traumatic tap will result in spillage of WBCs as well as RBCs into the peritoneal cavity. Correction should therefore be made for the presence of RBCs. For each 250 RBCs present, the PMN count must be reduced by one. The second mechanism is factitious elevation of the WBC count following diuresis. After diuresis, concentration of WBCs can occur since they are removed from the peritoneal space more slowly than fluid.[1,12] In order to make the diagnosis of a diuresis-induced elevation of the WBC count three conditions must be met: a normal pre-diuresis WBC count must be available, a predominance of lymphocytes must be present, and no unexplained clinical signs or symptoms may be present.[1] In uncomplicated ascites, PMNs should comprise approximately 25-30% of the WBC count, with the remainder predominantly lymphocytes. In spontaneous bacterial peritonitis (SBP), greater than 70% of the WBCs are PMNs.[1,2]

Albumin

Recent studies have demonstrated that calculation of the serum:ascites albumin gradient (SAAG) is an accurate diagnostic method for classifying the etiology of ascites.[5,19] This is calculated by subtracting the albumin content of the ascites from the serum albumin (both measured in gm/dL). A difference of greater than 1.1 g/dL is considered a high SAAG, with a difference of less than 1.1 g/dL reflecting a low SAAG. Portal hypertension is associated with a high SAAG and the gradient is considered approximately 97% accurate in diagnosing the presence or absence of portal hypertension.[1,2,4] The SAAG does not explain the etiology of the ascites; rather, it provides an accurate indication of portal pressure, and helps narrow the differential diagnosis of the etiology of the ascites. This calculation is considered accurate despite infection, paracentesis, diuresis and even albumin infusion.[1,2] The SAAG should replace the older terms of *transudate* and *exudate* when describing ascites. Specific diagnostic entities are associated with high and low SAAGs. High SAAG is associated with cirrhosis, alcoholic hepatitis, liver metastases, Budd-Chiari syndrome, congestive heart failure, portal vein thrombosis, veno-occlusive disease of the liver, fatty liver of pregnancy and myxedema.[1,2,7] Peritoneal carcinomatosis, tuberculous peritonitis, pancreatic ascites, bowel obstruction, nephrotic syndrome and connective tissue disease, conversely, are associated with a low SAAG.[1,2,7]

Microbiology

Recent studies have demonstrated that bedside inoculation of blood culture bottles with ascitic fluid is more sensitive than inoculation of agar plates with such fluid for the detection of bacterial infection.[13,14,15] Spontaneous bacterial peritonitis (SBP) is the most common infection of ascitic fluid.[2] Gram-negative rods are the most common infecting organisms, representing approximately 75% of cases.[9] *Escherichia coli* is isolated in approximately 50% of cases of gram-negative infection. Gram-positive cocci occur in approximately 25% of cases; *Streptococcus* species account for 70% of gram-positive isolates.[9] SBP is polymicrobial in a minority of cases (less than 10%). Anaerobic infection occurs in approximately 5% of cases.[9] In only slightly more than half of cases are blood cultures positive for the infecting organism.[9]

TECHNIQUE

Paracentesis should be performed using modified sterile technique. Gown and mask are considered optional, however sterile gloves, a sterile skin prep and sterile field are required.[6] Typically the patient is placed in the supine position, but if small amounts of ascites are present alternative positioning, such as a lateral, or rarely, a knee-hands position should be used. Ultrasound or CAT scan guidance may be used to localize small or loculated fluid collections. Drainage of the urinary bladder prior to performing the procedure is not required unless unusually distended.

Although lateral puncture sites have traditionally been felt to be the sites of choice, recent studies support the selection of a midline site two to three centimeters inferior to the umbilicus.[6,11,16] This is a generally avascular area. The skin should be cleansed with an appropriate disinfectant solution (povidone-iodine or chlorhexidine). If infection or a scar is present in the midline, a site several centimeters away should be chosen, preferably lateral to the rectus muscle.

Local anesthesia using 1% xylocaine in a Z-track method should be used. The Z-track technique involves retracting the skin inferiorly as the anesthetic and paracentesis needles are inserted. This creates a discontinuous path between the skin and subcutaneous tissues, decreasing the possibility of a persistent ascites leak. A wheal is created in the skin with the anesthetic, and then the skin is stretched creating the Z-track. The anesthesia needle is advanced slowly through the fascia and peritoneum, injecting the anesthetic agent in the process. When the peritoneum is entered, negative pressure through the syringe will generally result in a return of ascitic fluid into the syringe.

After anesthesia has been accomplished, the peritoneal cavity is accessed in a similar manner via the same Z-track. Single needle or catheter-over-needle techniques are the two predominant methods of paracentesis. In using the single needle technique, an 18 to 21 gauge needle is used to enter the peritoneum and withdraw the fluid. If the single needle technique is to be utilized just to obtain a small fluid specimen, some operators choose to forego the anesthesia. With the catheter-over-needle technique, the complete device is used to enter the peritoneum, the catheter is advanced and the needle withdrawn prior to removing fluid. Gentle aspiration of fluid through a 20-60 cc syringe may be used to remove small volumes of fluid or the needle/catheter may be connected to sterile tubing and larger volumes drained using gravity or suction bottles. Most operators prefer the catheter-over-needle method for removal of large volumes of fluid due to concerns over leaving a needle in the peritoneal cavity as the ascites is drained, fearing vascular or organ injury. However, single needle paracentesis has been done safely with the needle remaining in the peritoneum for more than an hour. [1] Potential disadvantages of the catheter-over-needle technique include shearing of the catheter into the peritoneum and kinking of the catheter with resultant obstruction to flow. Despite historical concerns over excessive fluid removal, recent studies have documented the safety of large volume paracentesis (over 5L).[1,3,4,8,] Cirrhotic patients with tense ascites undergoing repeated large volume paracentesis or total paracentesis should, however, be given albumin intravenously prior to the procedure, in an effort to help maintain an adequate intravascular volume.[4,8] Some patients develop irreversible renal and electrolyte abnormalities if they undergo large volume paracentesis without albumin infusion as a result of acute intravascular volume depletion.[8,17,18] If no fluid is returned after several attempts, ultrasound or CAT scan guidance can be used. At the conclusion of the procedure, withdraw the needle or catheter and apply an adhesive bandage to the puncture site.

COMPLICATIONS

Abdominal paracentesis is generally a benign procedure, with significant complications being quite unusual. Potential complications include small hematomas, hematomas requiring transfusion, fluid shifts with intravascular volume depletion, penetration of a solid or hollow viscus, iatrogenic peritonitis, and persistent fluid leak from the puncture site. As mentioned previously coagulopathy rarely results in significant complications. Small hematomas and hematomas requiring blood transfusion each have been reported to occur in less than one percent of patients.[10] Pretreatment with intravenous albumin minimizes the danger of intravascular volume depletion. Studies by Runyon revealed no incidents of iatrogenic peritonitis, hollow or solid viscus penetration, or death in more than 1000 paracenteses.[1,2] The risk of a continuous ascites leak is minimized by use of the Z-track method.

REFERENCES

1. Runyon BA. Ascites and spontaneous bacterial peritonitis. In Sleisenger MH, Fordtran JS, (eds): Gastrointestinal disease: pathophysiology, diagnosis, management. Philadelphia, WB Saunders, 5th edition, 1993, pp 1977-2003
2. Runyon BA. Ascites. In Schiff L, Schiff ER, (eds): Diseases of the liver. Philadelphia, JB Lippincott Co., 7th edition, 1993, pp 990-1015.
3. Carey WD. Ascites. In Achkar E, Farmer R, Fleshler B, (eds): Clinical Gastroenterology. Philadelphia, Lea and Febiger, 2nd edition, 1992, pp 106-117
4. Everson GT. Ascites in liver disease. In Levine J, (ed): Decision making in Gastroenterology. St. Louis, Mosby-Year Book, Inc., 2nd edition, 1992, pp 438-9
5. Rector WG, Reynolds TB. Superiority of serum-ascites albumin difference over the ascites total protein concentration in separation of "transudative" and "exudative" ascites. Am J Med 1984;77:83.
6. Lesesne HR. Abdominal paracentesis. In Drossman D, (ed): Manual of Gastroenterologic Procedures. Raven Press, New York, 3rd edition, 1993, pp 94-8.
7. Gerber DR, Bekes CE. Peritoneal catheterization. Critical Care Clinics 1992;8(4): 727-42.
8. Arroyo V, Gines P, Planas R. Treatment of ascites in cirrhosis. Gastroenterology Clinics in North America 1992;21(1):237-56.
9. Garcia-Tsao G. Spontaneous bacterial peritonitis. Gastroenterology Clinics in North America 1992;21(1):257-75.
10. Runyon BA. Paracentesis of ascitic fluid: A safe procedure. Arch Internal Med 1986;146:2259.
11. Bar-Meir S, Levner E, Conn HO. Analysis of ascitic fluid in cirrhosis. Dig Dis Sci 1979;24:136.
12. Hoefs JC: Increase in ascites WBC and protein concentrations during diuresis in patients with chronic liver disease. Hepatology 1981;1:249.
13. Bobadilla M, Sifuentes J, Garcia-Tsao G. Improved method for bacteriological diagnosis of spontaneous bacterial peritonitis. J Clin Microbiol 1989;27:2145.
14. Runyon BA. Ascitic fluid culture technique. Hepatology 1988;8:983.
15. Runyon BA, Umland ET, Merlin T. Inoculation of blood culture bottle with ascitic fluid: Improved detection of spontaneous bacterial peritonitis. Arch Internal Med 1987;147:73.

16. Mallory A, Schaefer JW. Complications of diagnostic paracentesis in patients with liver disease. JAMA 1978;239:628.
17. Gines P, Arroyo V, Quintero E, et al. Comparison of paracentesis and diuretics in the treatment of cirrhosis with tense ascites: Results of a randomized study. Gastroenterology 1987;93:234.
18. Gines P, Tito LI, Arroyo V, et al. Randomized comparative study of therapeutic paracentesis with and without intravenous albumin in cirrhosis. Gastroenterology 1988;94:1493.
19. Runyon BA, Montano AA, Akriviadis EA, Antillon MR, Irving MA, McHutchinson JG. Comparison of the utility of the serum-ascites albumin gradient to the exudate/transudate concept in the differential diagnosis of ascites. Hepatology 1992;16:85A.

NUTRITIONAL IMMUNOMODULATION IN SURGICAL PATIENTS

Brian J. Daley, M.D. and Collin E. M. Brathwaite, M.D.

University of Medicine and Dentistry of New Jersey
Robert Wood Johnson Medical School
Cooper Hospital/University Medical Center
Camden, New Jersey

The individual is protected from the microbiologic elements of his environment by a series of barriers. These include not only the skin, but also the respiratory and the gastrointestinal tracts. In addition to the physical barrier provided by the cornified epithelium of the skin, commensal skin flora and fatty acids secreted by the sebaceous glands help to prevent invasion of pathological organisms. Pathogens are usually prevented from gaining access to the respiratory tract by the mucociliary function of the upper airway epithelium and by the coughing (or sneezing) reflex. Those organisms that do gain access are usually eliminated by a variety of immunoglobulins secreted by the upper airway.

Of particular importance to the surgeon are the several mechanisms at work in the gastrointestinal tract which serve to protect the internal milieu of the host from invading organisms. Hydrochloric acid secreted in the stomach can effectively kill any ingested bacteria. This promotes a sterile environment in the stomach and the proximal small intestine. The continuous motion of peristalsis and metabolic activity of the bowel mucosa also serve as effective mechanisms by preventing stasis and bacterial overgrowth, and providing a protective barrier. The numerous pathogenic organisms in the colon and distal small bowel are prevented from gaining access by IgA antibodies contained in mucous secretions in these regions of the intestines. Additionally, the balance of the species of microorganisms within the bowel (colonization resistance) serves to prevent overgrowth and invasion of small pathogenic organisms.

Failure of the intestinal barrier due to bacterial overgrowth associated with bowel obstruction, malnutrition, loss of mucosal functional integrity due to severe hemorrhage, sepsis, or shock, can lead to pathogenic organisms gaining access to the systemic circulation via the lymph nodes or the portal circulation. This process has been termed bacterial translocation. It can result in profound immunologic consequences in the host.

Critical Issues in Surgery, Edited by A. C. Cernaianu et al.
Plenum Press, New York, 1995

The immune system of the patient is bolstered by a number of non-specific humoral mechanisms including the coagulation and the complement cascades. Cellular mechanisms are also integral parts of the immune defense. Phagocytic cells (macrophage and PMN's) and non-phagocytic cell-mediated immunity (macrophage/T-cell interaction and regulation of T-cell populations) play an important role. The system of mediators including cytokines, once released from the immune system cells, interact with receptors on target cells (which may be other immune cells, parenchymal cells, or vascular endothelial cells). The cytokine receptor interaction triggers a series of reactions in the immune system causing changes in secretory activity, change in receptor expression, and alteration in the structure of target cells. A detailed review of the humoral cell mediated and cytokine mechanisms of the immune system, may be found in any basic immunology text.

IMMUNE DYSFUNCTION

Injury, the stress of major surgery, and hemorrhage may cause significant alterations in the immune system to occur, placing the patient at risk for delayed septic complications. Indeed, the vast majority of late deaths after trauma and burns are due to sepsis.[1,2]

Neutrophils from injured patients have been shown to have depressed chemotaxis, phagocytosis, chemiluminescence, and intracellular killing.[3,4] In addition to reduced phagocytic activity of the reticuloendothelial system, due in part to reduced fibronectin levels and opsonic activity,[5] macrophages have reduced expression of Fc and C3b receptors after major hemorrhage.[6] This leads to reduced clearance of Fc and C3b complement products. Macrophages have also been shown to have impaired antigen presentation and altered cytokine production with elevated levels of interleukin-1 (IL-1), interleukin-6 (IL-6) and tumor necrosis factor (TNF) after hemorrhage.[7] These responses seem to occur early after hemorrhage. IL-1 and IL-6 levels peak at approximately 2 hours with IL-1 being cleared rapidly but IL-6 persisting for up to 24 hours.[8,9] Biologic activity of TNF is also absent by 24 hours.[10] Prostaglandin E_2 (PGE_2), a major immunosuppressive mediator, has also been shown to be significantly increased after hemorrhage.[11] In addition to several documented effects of PGE_2, it also causes a shift in the T-cell populations with decreased CD3 and CD4 subpopulations after hemorrhage.

Other lymphocyte responses to injury, hemorrhage, and surgical stress include loss of recall antigen responses or anergy, depression of B-cell or immunoglobulin production, increase in T-suppressor cell activity, decreased natural killer and lymphokine-activated killer cell activity, and production of immunosuppressive peptides.[12]

Several mechanisms may result in immunosuppression after accidental or surgical trauma. Surgical wounds or tissue destruction may result in the loss of functional integrity of the barrier systems resulting in pathogenic invasion of the internal milieu of the host. Devitalized tissue may then be responsible for local and systemic immumosuppressive effects. Breakdown of the barrier function of the gastrointestinal tract has been demonstrated in several animal studies[13,14] and in human studies.[15-17] Once bacterial translocation has occurred, it is believed that macrophage-derived cytokines and other mediators may cause systemic immunosuppression, and ultimately multiple organ dysfunction syndrome. The clinical relevance of bacterial translocation remains controversial. The neuroendocrine system which is also stimulated by injury also has an effect on the immune system resulting in impaired T-cell proliferation, immunoglobulin production, and reduced phagocytic activity.[18-20] Glucocorticoids and endorphins[21-24] have also been shown to affect the function of lymphocytes and phagocytic cells. Immunosuppressive humoral mediators including arachidonic acid metabolites have been found in the serum of injured patients. PGE_2 appears to be the most significant of these mediators. Inhibition of leukocyte chemotaxis has been linked to an 8 kd peptide identified in the serum of trauma patients.[4] Other suppressor factors including soluble receptors of TNF, IL-1, and IL-2 have been identified in circulation of injured patients. Suppressor cells ($CD8^+$ T-cells) have been seen in circulation after hemorrhage.[25] Tissue hypoxia and ischemia has been shown to reduce macrophage antigen presenting capabilities and also is associated with elevated TNF and PGE_2.[26] Finally, diminished nutritional intake in the face of major surgery or traumatic injury results in protein calorie malnutrition. Significant nitrogen losses occur. Aggressive nutritional support in this situation has been shown by several studies to correct the incidence of infectious complications.[27] The nutritional strategies available to the surgeon in managing these patients include preservation of normal host defenses by early aggressive metabolic and nutritional support, and immunologic stimulation via use of several agents that have been shown to have potential or definite pharmocologic effects on the immune system.

NUTRITIONAL PHARMOCOLOGIC AGENTS

In the past decade, significant interest has developed in the use of specific nutrients and growth factors aimed at correcting the immunologic pertubations that may follow injury or major surgery and reversing the severe catabolism of critical illness. The remainder of this chapter briefly describes our current knowledge of these immunonutrients.

Branch Chain Amino Acids

There have been recent reports that branch chain amino acids (BCAA)such as Leucine, Isoleucine, and Valine may improve nitrogen retention, increase lymphocyte count, improve plasma transferring levels, and reverse anergy to skin testing.[28] In a prospective randomized double blind trial of branch chain modified amino acid solutions, patients received standard amino acid solution, or BCAA-enriched formula as part of an isocaloric/isonitrogenous parenteral formula. BCAA-treated individuals had an elevated lymphocyte count from 800 to $1800/mm^3$ as well as improved nitrogen retention. (Table 1) Anergy to recall skin test antigens was reversed in 60% of the patients and plasma transferrin levels were improved in BCAA-treated individuals compared to controls. However, the conclusion from a subsequent research workshop sponsored by the American Society for Parenteral and Enteral Nutrition (ASPEN) was that… "in

Table 1. Branched Chain Amino Acid Effects

	Control Group		Branched Chain Amino Acid Group	
	Day 0	Day 7	Day 0	Day 7
Absolute lymphocyte count: (No./mm^3)	900 ± 38	1200 ± 600	800 ± 500	1800 ± 250*
Percent recall skin test positive	0	10	0	60†
Plasma transferrin	182 ± 32	186 ± 21	173 ±39	203 ±46*
Change in plasma transferrin from day 0 (mg/dL)		4.6 ± 28		31 ± 46*
Number of patients	11		12	

* = p<0.05; † = p<0.01; adapted from Cerra, et al.[28]

clinical studies, while some positive results in parameters of nitrogen metabolism have been noted using BCAA-enriched solutions in the more severely ill patients, little major effect on outcome has yet to be demonstrated."[29] Despite other clinical and laboratory studies suggesting improvement in nitrogen balance,[30,31] clinical outcome measures such as mortality have not been influenced.

Arginine

Arginine is a non-essential amino acid that is probably the most widely explored and best understood of the immunonutrients that have recently received great attention. After daily dietary supplements of 30 grams of arginine hydrochloride for 7 days, 21 healthy human volunteers were noted to have significantly increased stimulation indices of peripheral blood lymphocytes following concanavalin A (Con A) and phytohemagglutinin (PHA) stimulation.[32] Pharmacologic doses of arginine have also been shown to induce several biological responses including stimulation of pituitary growth hormone, insulin-like growth factor, prolactin, insulin, with a consequent improvement in wound healing.[33] Daly, et al. studied the immune and metabolic effects of arginine in a prospective randomized clinical trial in which postoperative surgical patients received 25 g/day of L-arginine supplementation or isonitrogenous L-glycine (43 g/day). T-lymphocyte response was significantly enhanced by day 7 after testing with Con A, PHA. CD4 (T-helper cell) expression was also significantly increased at day 7 in the arginine group.[34] (Figures 1, 2, 3) Other studies have documented the enhanced wound healing and lymphocyte response in humans after arginine supplementation.[35] Arginine is also a precursor for nitric oxide, a potent molecule resulting from the oxidation of the guanidine nitrogen of arginine, which is produced by a variety of cells including macrophages, neutrophils,neurons and vascular endothelial cells. Clearly, pharmacologic doses of arginine can enhance immune function and wound healing in both humans and animals. These functions are still being investigated, however arginine is now being supplemented in several commercial enteral formulas.

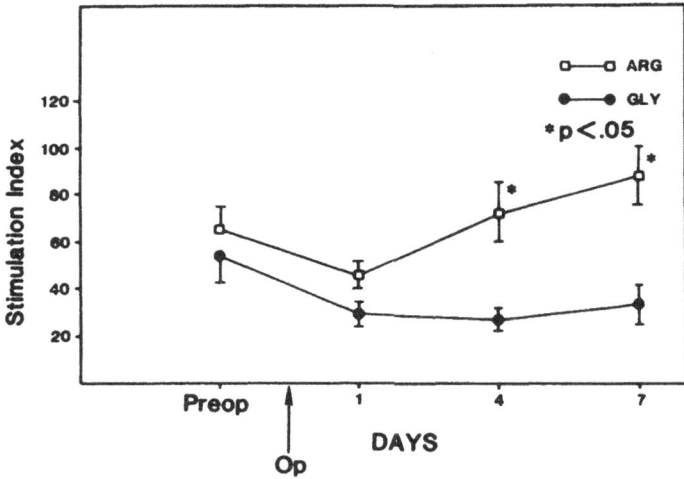

Figure 1. T lymphocyte activation. Conconavalin A (7 µg/mL).

Glutamine

Glutamine, the most abundant amino acid in the body, is generally considered to be non-essential in healthy humans. However, glutamine uptake by mucosal cells of the small intestines and immunologically active cells may exceed the rate of glutamine synthesis and release from the skeletal muscle during critical illness and thus render it essential under these circumstances. Glutamine serves a number of functions not the least of which is that it is the primary fuel source for enterocytes, lymphocytes and macrophages, and is important for maintaining renal acid-base status. Yoshida et al[36] have demon-

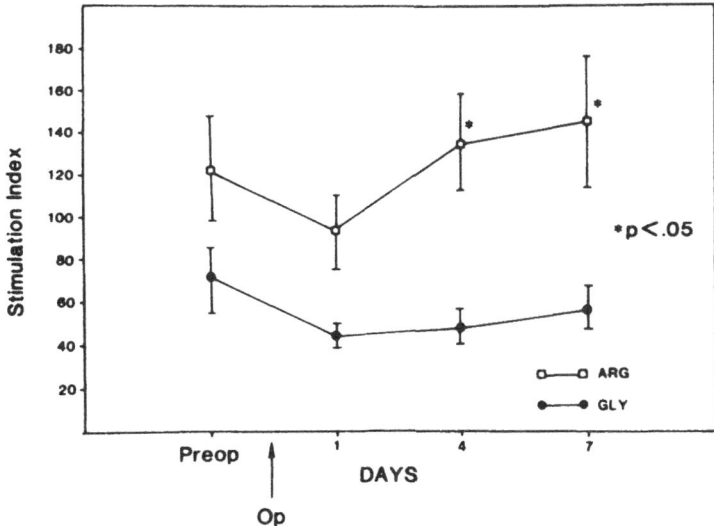

Figure 2. T lymphocyte activation. Phytohaemagglutinin (10 µg/mL).

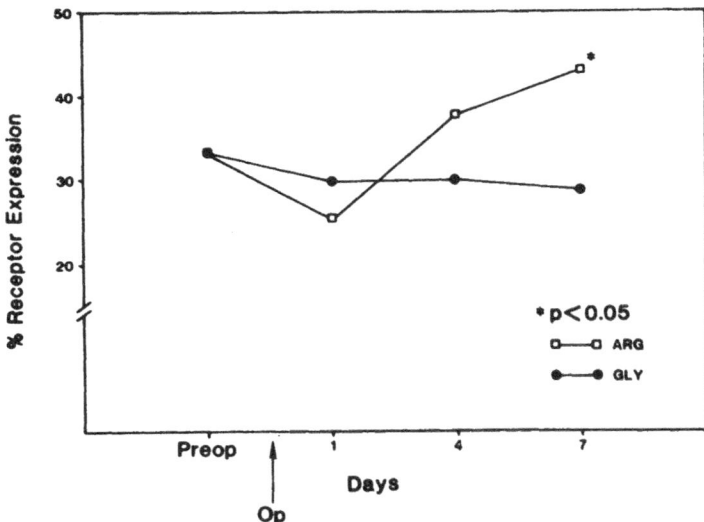

Figure 3. CD4 (T helper cell) expression.

strated improved small bowel mucosal functional integrity and architecture after glutamine supplementation in sepsis. Willmore, et al. have also demonstrated enhanced intestinal adaptation after massive small bowel resection with supplemental glutamine.[37] Other positive functions include reduction of bacterial translocation after radiation[38] as well as attenuation of intestinal and pancreatic atrophy associated with parenteral and enteral feeding.[39-41] In critically ill humans, D-xylose absorption, a measure of small bowel absorbative capacity, was shown to be enhanced by glutamine supplementation.[42] Additionally, in a study of allogeneic bone marrow transplantation with neutropenic patients, Ziegler, et al. demonstrated a decreased rate of infection, decreased microbial colonization of the stool, improved nitrogen balance, as well as reduction in length of stay in the hospital.[43] This has been the strongest evidence to date regarding the immunomodulatory effects of glutamine in hospitalized patients. However, despite these positive results, a large prospective randomized blinded trial looking strictly at the effects of glutamine supplementation is yet to be conducted.

Omega-3 Fatty Acids

The polyunsaturated fatty acids (PUFA) are a major component of cell membranes. The omega-6 family of PUFA which are derived from vegetable oils, form the major constituent in the membranes. Metabolites of omega-6 fatty acids, primarily PGE_2, inhibit cell mediated immune responses. Omega-6 fatty acids also inhibit natural killer cell activity, antibody formation, as well as release of some cytokines. The omega-3 fatty acids, major constituents of fish oils, generate eicosanoids with less biologic activity than the omega-6 PUFA. Dietary lipids in general are incorporated into the phospholipids of cell membranes with subsequent alteration in membrane functions including membrane receptor expression, cell-to-cell interactions, and cell signaling and cell surface enzyme activity.[44] Though the interactions between omega-3 and omega-6 fatty acids are rather complex, omega-3 fatty acids, after incorporation in macrophages stimulated with LPS, show reduced inositol phosphate production, dienoic eicosanoid release, and IL-1/TNF release.[45] In a prospective randomized blinded trial of a fish oil supplemented diet in patients undergoing major abdominal surgery, Kenler and colleagues noted a 50% decline in the total number of gastrointestinal complications, infections and positive cultures compared to controls.[46] The incorporation of omega-3 fatty acids into the diet has also been investigated in clinical trials involving combined nutrients and these will be discussed later.

Nucleotides

The synthesis of proteins depends on the production of RNA which itself depends on synthesis of the precursors, purines and pyrimidines. Dietary RNA, particularly uracil seems to be important for the normal maturational development of lymphocytes. The importance of RNA as a nutritional supplement has been investigated in studies involving nucleotide-free diets. Fanslow, et al. showed that mice maintained on a nucleotide free diet exhibited a significantly decreased mean survival time and a significantly increased rate of recovery of viable organisms in the spleen following intravenous injection of *candida albicans* compared to mice fed diets containing RNA or uracil as a nucleotide source.[47] (Figure 4) Although excess dietary sources of purines and pyrimidines are usually excreted, studies with nucleotide-free diets support additional dietary supplementation in conditions of metabolic stress.

Antioxidants (Vitamins A, C, E)

Since sepsis and organ injury are thought to be mediated by toxic oxygen species, antioxidants, play a potential role in controlling these

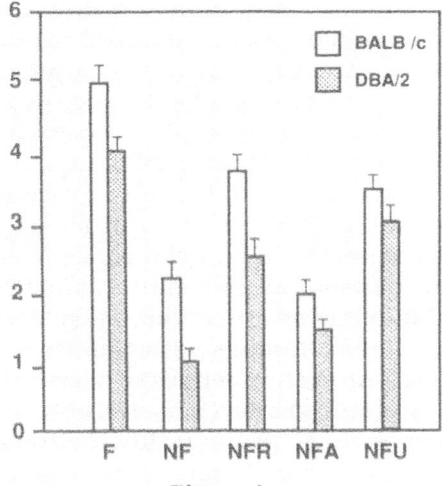

Figure 4

problems. Vitamins A, C and E have antioxidant properties and have been investigated in infected burned mice.[48] Mice treated with tocopherol daily before the burn had significantly lower mortality rates within controls, however, this protective effect was lost if tocopherol was not started until after the burn. None of the antioxidants in that study were effective when given after burn injury. Further studies are necessary to evaluate whether adjustment and treatment may offer some protection against immunosuppression of injured patients.

Growth Factors

Growth hormone is the most widely studied of the potential growth factors medically used. Herndon, et al. studied the effects of recombinant human growth hormone on wound healing in severely burned children.[49] These investigators noted a significantly decreased healing time of the donor site and decreased length of hospital stay in this study. Several authors have also demonstrated attenuated nitrogen losses after growth hormone supplementation in patients undergoing major surgical procedures.[50-52] Though insulin-like growth factor 1 is thought to be responsible for many of the functional effects of growth hormone, clinical trials have not yet been conducted.

Nutritional Immunomodulation-Combination Therapy

Though in-depth clinical trials with many of the nutrients outlined above have not yet been conducted, some of the substances have been combined and studied in the critically ill or post-surgical patients. Alexander and Gottschlich conducted a prospective randomized study in 60 burn patients.[53] Patients were randomized to an experimental diet containing elevated omega-3 fatty acids, omega-6 fatty acids as well as increased arginine versus a control diet (Osmolyte or Traumacal). These investigators noted a 75% less wound infection rate and a 31% reduction in length of stay in the experimental group. In a subsequent study, Daly et al conducted a prospective randomized double-blind study in 85 patients after major upper gastrointestinal surgery.[54] The experimental group in this study received a commercially prepared product Impact® (Sandoz Nutrition, Minneapolis, MN) while controls received Osmolyte HN® (Ross Laboratories). Impact® contains pharmacologic supplementation of omega-3 fatty acids, arginine, and RNA. This study noted a 73% reduction in incidence of infection and wound complications and a 22% reduction in length of stay in the study group. The study was conducted in surgical patients who underwent major resection of upper gastrointestinal tract cancer. Most recently in a prospective randomized double-blind multi-center study involving ICU patients, Bower, et al. reported similar findings with Impact.®[55] Septic patients fed Impact® had a reduction in median length of hospital stay of 10 days and significant reduction in acquired infections. Notably, however, there was no difference in nitrogen balance or mortality between experimental and control groups. Additionally, in a climate of managed care, the interpretation of hospital length of stay data is controversial.

Route of Feeding

The route of feeding may have immunologic effects on the immune system. This has been investigated in numerous reports with conflicting results in generally small groups of patients. The conclusion of more recent studies appears to be that the preferred route for provision of nutritional support particularly in the critically ill patient is the enteral route. It is more physiologic in terms of nutrient utilization, is considerably less expensive than parenteral nutrition, and current evidence suggests that it can significantly reduce the incidence of infectious complications in critically ill humans especially when provided early.[56,57]

REFERENCES

1. Baker CC, Oppenheimer L, Stevens B, et al. Epidemiology of trauma deaths. Am J Surg 1980;140:144.
2. Polk HC. Consensus summary on infection. J Trauma 1979;19:894-896.
3. Martin TR, Pistorese BP, Hudson LD, et al. The function of lung and blood neutrophils in patients with the adult respiratory distress syndrome. Am Rev Respir Dis 1991;14:254-262.
4. Christou MV, Meakins JL. Partial analysis and purification of polymorphonuclear neutrophil chemotactic inhibitors in serum from anergic patients. Arch Surg 1983;18:156-160.
5. Saba TM, Lanser ME, Dillon BC. Opsonic fibronectin and phagocytic defense after trauma. In: Handbook of shock and trauma, Vol 1. Basic Science. Altura BM, Lefer AM, Shumer W (eds). New York, Raven Press, 1983, pp 167-181.
6. Ayala A, Perrin MM, Wagner MA, et al. Enhanced susceptibility to sepsis following simple hemorrhage. Depression of Fc and C3b receptor mediated phagocytosis. Arch Surg 1990;125:70-75.
7. Ayala A, Perrin MM, Chaudry IH. Defective macrophage antigen presentation following hemorrhage is associated with the loss of MHC class II (Ia) antigens. Immunology 1990;70:33-39.
8. Abraham E, Richmond JN, Chang YH. Effects of hemorrhage on interleukin 1 production. Circ Shock 1988;25:33-40.
9. Ayala A, Perrin MM, Ertel W, et al. Differential effects of hemorrhage on Kupffer cells. Decreased antigen presentation despite increased inflammatory cytokines (IL-1, IL-6 and TNF) release. Cytokine 1992;4:66-75.
10. Ayala A, Perrin MM, Meldrum DR, et al. Hemorrhage induces an increase in serum TNF which is not associated with elevated levels of endotoxin. Cytokine 1990;2:170-174.
11. Ertel W, Morrison MH, Ayala A, et al. Anti-TNF monoclonal antibodies prevent hemorrhage induced suppression of Kupffer cell antigen presentation and MHC class II antigen expression. Immunology 1991;74:290-297.
12. Ninnemann JL. The immune consequences of trauma: An overview. In: Immune consequences of trauma, shock and sepsis. Faist E, Ninnemann J, Green D (eds). Springer-Verlag, Berlin, 1989, pp 1-8.
13. Baker JW, Deitch EA, Li M, et al. Hemorrhagic shock induces bacterial translocation from the gut. J Trauma 1988;28:896-906.
14. Deitch EA, Bridges W, Baker J, et al. Hemorrhagic shock-induced bacterial translocation is reduced by xanthine oxidase inhibition or inactivation. Surgery 1988;104:191-198.
15. Brathwaite CEM, Ross SE, Nagele R, et al. Significance of bacterial translocation after multiple trauma with hemorrhagic shock. Circ Shock 1992;37:50.
16. Brathwaite CEM, Ross SE, Nagele R, et al. Bacterial translocation occurs in humans after traumatic injury: Evidence using immunofluorescence. J Trauma 1993;34:586-590.

17. Reed L, Martin M, Manglano R, et al. Bacterial translocation following abdominal trauma in humans. Circ Shock 1994;42:1-6.

18. Crary B, Borysenko M, Sutherland DC, et al. Decrease in mitogen responsiveness of mononuclear cells from peripheral blood after epinephrine administration in humans. J Immunol 1983;130:694-697.

19. Feldman RD, Hunninghake GW, McArdle WL. Beta adrenergic receptor-mediated suppression of interleukin 2 receptors in human lymphocytes. J Immunol 1987;139:3355-3359.

20. Loegering DJ, Commins LM. Effect of beta receptor stimulation on Kupffer cell complement receptor clearance function. Circ Shock 1988;25:325-332.

21. Clayman HN. Corticosteroid and lymphoid cells. N Engl J Med 1972;287:388-397.

22. Gillis S, Crabtree GR, Smith KA. Glucocorticoid-induced inhibition of T-cell growth factor production. The effect on mitogen induced lymphocyte proliferation. J Immunol 1979;123:1624-1631.

23. Snyder DS, Unanue ER. Corticosteroids inhibit murine macrophage Ia expression and interleukin production. J Immunol 1982;129:1803-1805.

24. Deitch EA, Xu D, Bridges RM. Opioids modulate human neutrophil and lymphocyte function: Thermal injury alters plasma beta endorphin levels. Surgery 1988;104:41-48.

25. Abraham E, Chang YH. Generation of functionally active suppressor cells by hemorrhage and hemorrhagic serum. Clin Exp Immunol 1988;72:238-242.

26. Morrison MH, Ertel W, Ayala A, et al. Depressed antigen presentation of peritoneal macrophage following hypoxia is associated with altered release of inflammatory mediators. FASEB J 1992;6(A):1614.

27. Alexander JW, McMillan BG, Stinnett JD, et al. Beneficial effects of progressive protein feeding in severely burned children. Ann Surg 1980;192:505-517.

28. Cerra FB, Mazuski JE, Chute E, et al. Branched chain metabolic support: A prospective randomized double blind trial in surgical stress. Ann Surg 1984;199:286-291.

29. Brennan M, Cerra FB, Daly JM, et al. Report of a research workshop: Branched chain amino-acid in stress and injury. J Parenter Enteral Nutr 1986;10:446-452.

30. Delany HM, Teh E, Dwarka B, et al. Infusion of enteral vs. parenteral nutrients using high-concentration branch-chain amino acids: Effect on wound healing in postoperative rat. J Parenter Enteral Nutr 1991;15:464-468.

31. Okada A, Mori S, Totsuka M, et al. Branched-chain amino acids metabolic support in surgical patients: A randomized, controlled trial in patients with subtotal or total gastrectomy in 16 Japanese institutions. J Parenter Enteral Nutr 1988;12:332.

32. Barbul A, Sisto D, et al. Arginine stimulates lymphocyte immune response in healthy human beings. Surgery 1981;90:244-251.

33. Barbul A. Arginine: Biochemistry, physiology and therapeutic implications. J Parenter Enteral Nutr 1986;10:227-238.

34. Daly JM, Reynolds JV, Thom A, et al. Immune and metabolic effects of arginine in the surgical patient. Ann Surg 1988;208:512-23.

35. Barbul A, Lazarou SA, Efron DT, et al. Arginine enhances wound healing and lymphocyte response in humans. Surgery 1990;108:331-7.

36. Yoshida S, Leskiw MJ, Schluter MD, et al. Effect of total parenteral nutrition, systemic sepsis, and glutamine on gut mucosa in rats. Am J Physiol 1992;263:368-73.

37. Wilmore DW, Smith RJ, O'Dwyer ST, et al. The gut: A central organ after surgical stress. Surgery 1988;104:917-23.

38. Souba WW, Klimberg VS, Hautamaki RD, et al. Oral glutamine reduces bacterial translocation following abdominal radiation. J Surg Res 1990;48:1-5.

39. O'Dwyer SO, Smith RJ, Swang TL, et al. Maintenance of small bowel mucosa with glutamine enriched parenteral nutrition. J Parenter Enteral Nutr 1989;13:579-85.

40. Jacobs DO, Evans DA, Mealy K, et al. Combined effects of glutamine and epidermal growth factor on the rat intestine. Surgery 1988;104:358-64.

41. Helton WS, Jacobs DO, Bonner-Weir S, et al. Effects of glutamine-enriched parenteral nutrition on the exocrine pancreas. J Parenter Enteral Nutr 1990;14:344-52.

42. Tremel H, Kienle B, Weilemann LS, et al. Glutamine dipeptide supplemented TPN maintains intestinal function in the critically ill. Clin Nutr 1992;1125.

43. Zeigler TR, Young LS, Benfell K, et al. Clinical and metabolic efficacy of glutamine supplemented parenteral nutrition after bone marrow transplantation: A randomized, double-blind controlled study. Ann Intern Med 1992;116:821.
44. Kinsella JE, Lokesh B, Broughton S, Whelan J. Dietary polyunsaturated fatty acids and eicosanoids: Potential effects on the modulation of inflammatory and immune cells. An overview. Nutrition 1990;6:24-44.
45. Billar TR, Bankey PE, Svingen BA, et al. Fatty acid intake and Kupffer cell function: Fish oil alters eicosanoid and monokine production to endotoxin stimulation. Surgery 1988;104:343-348.
46. Kenler A, Swails W, Driscoll D, Daley B, et al. Early enteral feeding in post surgical cancer patients: Fish oil structured lipid-based polymenic formula versus a standard polymenic formula. Submitted for publication.
47. Fanslow WC, Kulkarni A, Van Buren C, Rudolph F. Effect of nucleotide restriction and supplementation on resistance to experimental murine candidiasis. J Parenter Enteral Nutr 1988;12;49-52.
48. Fang C, Peck MD, Alexander JW, et al. The effect of free radical scavengers on outcome after infection in burned mice. J Trauma 1990;30:453-456.
49. Herndon DN, Barrow RE, Kunkel KR, et al. Effects of recombinant human growth hormone on donor-site healing in severely burned children. Ann Surg 1990;212:424-31.
50. Jiang Z, He G, Zhang S, et al. Low dose growth hormone and hypocaloric nutrition attenuate the protein-catabolic response after major operation. Ann Surg 1989;210:513-25.
51. Ponting GA, Halliday D, Teale JD, Sim AJW. Postoperative positive nitrogen balance with intravenous hyponutrition and growth hormone. Lancet 1988;I:438-40.
52. Ward HC, Halliday D, Sim AJW. Protein and energy metabolism with biosynthetic human growth hormone after gastrointestinal surgery. Ann Surg 1987;206:56-61.
53. Alexander JW, Gottschlich MM. Nutritional immunomodulators in burn patients. J Crit Care Med 1990;18:149-153.
54. Daly JM, Lieberman MD, Goldfine J, et al. Enteral nutrition with supplemental arginine, RNA, and omega-3 fatty acids in patients after operation: Immunologic, metabolic, and clinical outcome. Surgery 1992:112:56-67.
55. Bower R, Cerra F, Bershadsky B, et al. Early enteral administration of a formula (Impact®)supplemented with arginine, nucleotides, and fish oil in intensive care unit patients: Results of a multicenter, prospective, randomized, clinical trial. Crit Care Med 1995;23:436-449.
56. Moore FA, Feliciano DV, Andrassy RJ, et al. Early enteral feeding, compared with parenteral, reduces postoperative septic complications: The results of a meta-analysis. Ann Surg 1991;216:172-83.
57. Kudsk KA, Croce MA, Fabian TC, et al. Enteral versus parenteral feeding: Effects on septic morbidity after blunt and penetrating abdominal trauma. Ann Surg 1992;215:503-513.

PHYSICIAN ASSISTANTS: AN OVERVIEW

John F. Byrnes, Jr., PA-C

Southeastern Clinical Services
Orlando, Florida

The year 1993 marked the 25th anniversary of the first practicing physician assistant (PA), following graduation from the inaugural program at Duke University. From the entering class of 1965, over 25,000 active practicing PAs have graduated from 55 PA programs throughout the United States. Prime projections indicate a need for an additional 10,000 to 15,000 PAs by the year 2000, and an additional 25 to 30 PA programs during the same time span. Funding has just been increased to enlarge the number of students accepted into the current programs, and a reduction in physician-specialty residency slots over the next three or four years will result in an increase in need for mid-level providers, such as PAs.

Over a third of all practicing PAs work in areas of population sizes of less than 50,000 people, and an additional 22 percent of all PAs work in population bases ranging from 50,000 to 250,000 people (Table 1).

PAs are skilled members of the health care team who practice medicine with the supervision of licensed physicians, filling a broad range of medical services that would otherwise be provided by a physician. Table 2 presents common PAs responsibilities. These include history and physical examinations, ordering laboratory and diagnostic tests, patient management plans (including the writings of prescriptions), charting patient information, patient counseling and information dispensing, and medical and surgical therapeutic procedures.

The education for PAs average two years in length with the first year consisting of didactic training followed by a second year of clinical rotations. The didactic training is similar to many of the courses taken in the first year of medical school, and clinical rotations are taken in conjunction with fourth year medical students, along with residents in teaching programs. Approximately 1,400 students graduate annually from the 55 accredited programs. The prerequisites for acceptance into PA programs include a minimum of a 2-year college degree, although most applicants have a 4-year degree before enrolling. Additionally, at least one year of clinical experience in a health-related field, along with recommendations from peers and medical supervising personnel is required.

Critical Issues in Surgery, Edited by A. C. Cernaianu et al.
Plenum Press, New York, 1995

Table 1. Distribution of Physician
Assistants by Community Size

Population	Percent
< 5,000	8.7
5–10,000	8.7
10–50,000	16.1
50–250,000	21.9
250–500,000	11.4
500–1,000,000	12.9
> 1,000,000	20.1

In 1967, Dr. John Kirklin started the first Surgeon Assistant (SA) program at the University of Alabama, and there are three current SA programs in existence today. They include the program at the University of Alabama, along with Cornell University, and Cuyahoga Community College. There are over 4,000 graduates of SA and PA programs currently working in surgical specialties. Although the clinical rotations undertaken in SA programs are entirely surgical rotations, the national boards remain the same for SA and PA program graduates, and the job roles and responsibilities are similar following graduation, regardless of the type of program from which the PA graduated.

While the original emphasis for the development of physician assistants was to provide primary care services in underserved areas, specialization has not escaped what most consider to be a natural evolution of a growing field of medical providers. In 1974, approximately 20 percent of PA's were in surgical positions; 1990 found the present average of almost 30 percent of practicing PAs employed in surgical specialty areas (Table 3).

A definition of what constitutes a qualified assistant in surgery was written by the American Academy of Physician Assistants, in conjunction with the American College of Surgeons and the Association of Operating

Table 2. Role of the Surgical Physician Assistant

Admission history and physical exam; discharge summaries
Rounds, progress notes pre/post operative orders
Convey verbal orders from physicians to nursing staff
Maintain certification,
Initiate emergency measures
    Endotracheal intubation
    Cardiac defibrillation
    Administration of iv medications
Surgical assisting
Postoperative wound care
Removal of devices
    Chest tubes
    Hemodynamic monitoring catheters
    Temporary pacing wires
Review of medical records
On-call status as required
Research

ACLS = Advanced coronary life support
Source: 1993 American Academy of Physician Assistant Census.

Table 3. Physician Assistants by Specialty

Specialty	Percent
Internal Medicine	9.0
Internal Medicine Subspecialty	6.0
Industrial Occupational Medicine	3.5
OB/GYN	3.0
Geriatrics	1.2
Emergency Medicine	8.5
General Pediatrics	2.3
Pediatric Subspecialty	1.0
General Surgery	7.1
Surgical Subspecialty	10.0
Orthopedics	8.0
Other Specialties	8.0
Family General Practice	33.0

Source: 1993 American Academy of
Physician Assistant Census.

Room Nurses. This definition states that a qualified assistant in surgery should have:

1. Manual dexterity and technical proficiency,
2. In-depth knowledge of surgical asepsis, anatomy, physiology and operative technique related to the specific procedures,
3. Sufficient education and training to make the appropriate intra-operative decisions concerning the care of the patient and progress of the intended procedure should the surgeon be unable to complete the procedure.

The training of a surgical PA encompasses all three of the above recommended requirements for a qualified assistant in surgery. In this capacity, the PA does provide a very cost-effective and qualified assistant in the surgical arena.

Acceptance of PAs into the health care profession has increased dramatically since 1957, as PAs have been found to be generally more accessible than their employing physicians; they provide a good liaison between nursing and physicians when the physicians are not available. In a combined physician-PA practice, more time can be spent with the team approach to the care of the patient. Additionally, PAs allow physicians more discretionary time.

Currently, there is widespread acceptance amongst hospitals and medical staffs in utilization of PAs in a wide diversity of areas. Many hospitals are employing PAs directly to provide services that were performed previously by residents, in situations where teaching positions have been eliminated due to cost control measures. PAs are certified or licensed in all 50 states, including the District of Columbia and Guam. Following initial certification upon completion of the PA program, each PA is required to accumulate 100 hours of Continuing Medical Education every two years, along with a re-certification process every six years. The re-certification process can be either a proctored examination, or a series of modules selected to encompass the specific responsibilities of a PA in a specialty setting.

Table 4. Physician Assistant Employment Setting

Federal, State, Local Governments, Armed Forces	17.8%
Hospitals	28.0%
Group/Solo Practices	42.3%
HMO	7.3%
Rural Clinics	5.1%
Inner City Clinics	1.2%
Other	5.0%

Many physician organizations have established liaisons with PA organizations, such as the American College of Surgeons (ACS), the American Association of Surgeons Assistants (AASA), the American Association of Thoracic Surgeons (AATS), and the American Association of Physician Assistants in Cardiovascular Surgery (APACVS). Additionally, liaisons are being explored between the PA specialty groups in neurosurgery, orthopedics, OB/GYN, ENT, and emergency medicine to respective physician counterpart organizations.

PAs are employed in almost every conceivable medical setting, including the Armed Forces and government agencies. While approximately 18 percent of PAs are employed by the government, the remainder of the PAs are employed in hospitals, groups of specialized practices, HMO's, and other settings as seen in Table 4.

PA services are covered by most third-party carriers, as well as the federal government through Medicare and CHAMPUS reimbursement programs. Since 1986, PAs have been reimbursed by Medicare at a rate of 65 percent of the prevailing physician's rate for surgical assisting, 75 percent for hospital services/procedures, 85 percent for nursing home care, and 100 percent for federally designated manpower health shortage areas. Many HMOs and health care plans are offering provider status to PAs, and current legislation pending before Congress proposes raising the rate of reimbursement for PA services under the Medicare guidelines (Table 5).

Prescriptive practice authority is provided to PAs in 32 states, the District of Columbia and Guam. Most in-patient settings in all 50 states

Table 5. Physician Assistants Reimbursement

Salary ($)	Percent
< 40,000	17.0
40–50,000	35.5
50–60,000	23.6
60–70,000	11.5
70–80,000	5.9
80–90,000	2.9
90–100,000	1.7
> 100,000	2.0
Average	53,500

Source: 1993 American Association
of Physician Assistant Census

allow PAs to order prescriptive medication for their patients under the supervision of their physician. Prescriptive practice regulations mentioned here pertain to out-patient settings. Some of the states that allow PAs prescriptive practice have positive and/or negative formularies, but the addition of this very important responsibility has increased the effectiveness of having a PA in a practice setting.

Medical malpractice premiums for PAs are very minimal, and many are riders attached to the employing surgeon's policy. Law suits against individual PAs are almost nonexistent without their employing physician or institution also being involved, and the monetary amount of the claims has been, to date, very minimal.

The future provides many opportunities for PA and their employing physicians. Fields such as cardiac surgery, neurosurgery, transplant surgery, and trauma surgery that require high tech procedures and highly trained personnel can only benefit from this rapidly growing and cost-effective health care provider.

PHYSICIANS ASSISTANTS: A COST-EFFICIENT SOLUTION FOR THE SURGICAL PRACTICE

Linda A. Garry, PA-C and Debra L. Priore, PA-C

University of Medicine and Dentistry of New Jersey
Robert Wood Johnson Medical School
Cooper Hospital/University Medical Center
Camden, New Jersey

Since the advent of the first medical specialty in the 1860's, Americans have witnessed a proliferation of the number and types of medical specialties and subspecialties. The role of the Physician Assistant (PA) has changed during the last 25 years. Today's Physician Assistant is involved in every aspect of health care and needs provision, expanding and diversifying into a multitude of subspecialized areas. Both physicians and PAs have been moving away from the early generalist tradition.

Surgical specialties have been a rapidly growing segment of PA employment. In 1974, approximately 19 percent of PAs practiced in the surgical field. By 1993, this number has increased to 28 percent. The expansion of opportunities for surgical PAs is the result of both cutbacks in many surgical residency programs and national restrictions on the employment of foreign medical graduates. Surgical PAs can fill the need for house staff in those hospitals without residents.

In 1886, Dr. Howard Lilenthal became the first formally trained physician to elect specialization in a field other than general medicine. Dr. Lilenthal, an intern at Mt. Sinai Hospital in New York, chose surgery over medicine, establishing the option for a post graduate trained physician to select a specialization or consulting practice. Ophthalmology became the first organized specialty in 1916. By contrast, it took only 2 years from the inception of the first general PA at Duke University in 1965, to the establishment of a PA specialty program. The first surgeon's assistant program began in 1967; and others soon followed. The first post graduate PA program, in surgery, at Montefiore Hospital Bronx, New York was followed by a similar program at Norwalk Hospital and Yale University Medical Center in Connecticut in 1976.

PAs are an integral part of the surgical team, providing coordinated, consistent, and comprehensive care. In addition to the technical aspects

Critical Issues in Surgery, Edited by A. C. Cernaianu et al.
Plenum Press, New York, 1995

provided to patients, PAs are able to continually incorporate patient and family counseling and education into a comprehensive plan of care.

In a busy surgical practice, the PA can be a valuable asset providing time-efficient and cost-effective health care services. An outpatient surgical PA can work in and is interchangeable in all fields of surgical specialty. PA's obtain complete patient histories and perform physical examinations. If patients are undergoing surgery, the PA can provide all the necessary educational and pre-admission information. Patients are made aware of the easy availability of the PA if any questions or concerns about their care should arise. At the initial office visit, the surgeon saves time since histories, physical examinations, progress notes, and most necessary paper work are completed by the PA. Patients report feeling more comfortable knowing there is a liaison between themselves and the surgeon.

In post-operative care, PA's provide information on wound and pain management. Patients see the PA for control of wound healing, suture and staple removal, or any other problems related to the postoperative period. This helps the surgical practice, since the surgeon can spend more time on other complex problems. An important aspect in a surgical practice is to return patient's phone calls promptly. The PA can return phone calls and quickly answer questions, reassure patients, relay test results, and renew prescriptions. This helps to alleviate patient's anxiety and reduces the work load for the surgeon.

PA's are strong advocates of preventive medicine. With the inception of screening programs by PA's in a surgical practice, early detection of breast and colorectal cancers have been made possible. PA's can perform and teach breast self-examinations and recommend age-appropriate guidelines. They may perform digital rectal examinations, test for blood in the stool, perform flexible sigmoidoscopies and explain guidelines for colorectal health. PA,s may also initiate smoking cessation programs in a surgical practice, promote healthy lifestyle changes and thereby decrease patient's risk for potential cardiac and vascular problems.

Good public relations are important for a surgical group since it can increase patient volume. PA's can provide community outreach programs i.e. public awareness of breast and colorectal health. Moreover, the PA may be involved in research. A PA can recruit and screen patients for research studies, obtain data and improve the effectiveness of such studies. They may also be involved in the writing of scientific communications as well as obtaining needed medical information quickly from charts, patients, or from the literature.

PA's are a vital force in the health care system. They increase efficiency within a surgical practice, reduce patient waiting time, allow physicians more time for difficult cases, bring a team approach to the practice, help support staff and, above all, contribute to providing optimal patient care.

The demand for PAs has dramatically increased over the years and the current demand for PAs far exceeds the available supply. There is also and increased awareness of PA's educational background and capabilities. There are currently 7 jobs for every PA and this ratio significantly increases if the PA has chosen a specialty, such as surgery.

As a result, PA's salaries have increased in the past few years and are becoming highly competitive. It is important to remember, nonetheless, that

PAs will always be a cost efficient way to provide health care since the surgeon may bill for services rendered by the PA. Unlike physicians, surgical PAs have a limited career mobility. Adjustments must be made to provide appropriate scheduling, compensation and training to accommodate the surgical PA's permanent employment situation. A commitment must be made to provide surgical PAs the support, supervision and continuing education appropriate to their profession and their function as members of the surgical team.

The PA profession has demonstrated its ability to adapt to a constantly changing health care environment. PAs have been able to pursue ideas with their particular practice settings according to their individual skills and interests and have contributed to the professional growth and development of the physician assistant profession, making significant contributions to meeting the nation's health care needs.

SUGGESTED READING

Brandt B, Beinfield MS, Laffoye HA, Baue AE: The training and utilization of surgical physician assistants. Arch Surg 1989, 124:348–353.
Rothwell P: PAs in cardiothoracic surgery. J Am Acad Phys Assist 1993;6:150-7

FUTURE 2000 FOR NURSES

Zane Robinson Wolf, PhD, RN

LaSalle University Albert Einstein Medical Center
Philadelphia, Pennsylvania

The rigors and the advantages of the nursing profession are presently of great interest to the public which is more aware than ever of the many roles that nurses play in the American health care delivery system. Furthermore, a possible nursing shortage and the economic recession made possible to induce greater numbers of women and men to consider nursing as a career. All who choose nursing and practice in the context of the fact and fiction about the profession face the future together.

Part of the *Future 2000* is predictable for nurses who are continuing on or just beginning their professional careers; some trends are already in the making. These include efforts to establish collaborative practices between nurses and physicians, consultative practices owned by nurse entrepreneurs, competitive marketplace ventures spearheaded by nurse entrepreneurs, direct reimbursement of nursing practice, and more creative and influential input into social policy decisions. In the next few years, events will shape these trends. This chapter will examine some of the emerging trends in the nursing profession.

ENTREPRENEURS AND INTRAPRENEURS: DREAMERS OF DESIGNER DREAMS AND BLENDERS OF AUTONOMY AND ALTRUISM

Nurse intrapreneurs employed by the health care institutions will continue to expand their practice spheres within current institutional boundaries. They will capitalize on their skills by valuing their professional competence, and develop a more appreciative regard for what they know, what they can do, what they value, and pool their expertise by developing consultative services for patients and physicians. They will design, carry out, use, and benefit from behavioral research, since it is already certain that behavioral factors or lifestyle contribute to the burden of illness. Some of the burden is associated with cigarette smoking, consumption of alcoholic beverages, illicit drugs, dietary habits, insufficient exercise, and maladap-

Critical Issues in Surgery, Edited by A. C. Cernaianu et al.
Plenum Press, New York, 1995

tive responses to social pressures. Nurses have created and participated in programs to address these issues. They will continue to reach out to the larger community in order to offer options for people to change their behavior.

Nurse entrepreneurs will join in competitive ventures in the health marketplace by developing and marketing new services for ambulatory care settings, home health care agencies, personal care home, occupational health, and school settings. They are already aware of the influences of chronic illness and the lengthening life spans on consumption of part of the gross national product that encompasses health care services. Nurse entrepreneurs will teach personal care skills as well as high and low tech skill to nurses and family members. They will encourage them to manage stress and resolve conflict. Some examples of entrepreneurial efforts include intravenous therapies at home, enterostomal therapy, family planning, and midlife women's health counselling. Extensive experience in the practice field, currency in practice, competence, and clinical scholarship will make entrepreneurial and intrapreneurial services indispensable. Both experts will continue to network through professional nursing and other professional groups.

THE CARE/CURE CONNECTION THROUGH COLLABORATION: TOWARD A NEW WORLD ORDER

Presently, the relationship between American nurses and physicians is not a collaborative one at present. In spite of the wishes of many nurses, collaborative efforts falter between both groups of health care providers. As nurses feel increasingly comfortable with their altruistic motives and autonomous behaviors, they are establishing themselves as care givers to be reckoned with. However, many physicians and other professionals fail to include nurses when multi-disciplinary conferences are called and when problems involving both groups are discussed. Consequently, nurses strain at the paternalism that pervades the hierarchical health care system that thrives in American hospitals and other health care agencies. They hope for better days when nurses and physicians work together for better patient outcomes.

Some physicians may not appreciate the efforts of nurses to establish autonomous practice. They are confused and yearn for the good old days when head nurses met physicians at the door of units, charts in hand, and accompanied physicians on their rounds. Some physicians resent that nurses and physicians record patient data on the same progress notes on hospital charts. However, some nurses and physicians manage to work together in collaborative practices. In these situations, nurses are treated like equals and receive salaries equivalent with their responsibilities.

There is hope. A few universities have developed collaborative practice courses during which senior, baccalaureate nursing and medical students learn together. These courses join the literature that exhorts both groups to work together in order to pass the nurse-doctor game, the anger, and the confusion in order to improve patient care outcomes.

There is another collaborative effort that needs attention. Nursing education and nursing practice must continue their efforts to blend the academic world and the clinical practice. All nurses have to realize that, even though the corporate world of the university and the health care agency address different missions, many of their goals are similar.

The separation of education and practice that took place when nursing education moved into higher education can no longer persist. Both, education and practice are in ideal positions to network now in order to achieve mutually desirable goals. Some have begun to work on convergent goals by creating a regional planning agency to address the nursing shortage problem and by establishing joint ventures through joint appointments and reverse joint appointments. Another way that collaborative efforts will pay off is through adjunct appointments in schools of nursing of nurses employed health care agencies. Both sides benefit. Clinicians, managers, and administrators teach what they enjoy and are listed as adjunct faculty and students see nurses who are *real* nurses. Exchanges may also take place through mentor programs where nursing students meet with clinicians and see them working, testing their ideas of what nurses do at work. Finally, some nurses are reaching out to share research expertise. The Tri-State Nursing Research Consortium was begun by Dr. Suzanne Langner, at the Graduate Hospital in Philadelphia. Nurses from many health care agencies and universities meet initially in small groups to determine if they can join research efforts and network to share ideas. Recently attendance has dwindled. Benefits from these previous examples of collaboration will move nurses in to the future and a new world order.

EMERGING CLINICAL SCHOLARSHIP

Clinical scholarship, based on the knowledge and learning derived from analytic observations of clients and patients, has a long tradition in American nursing. This concept has developed slowly over the past century and has been shaped by nurses examining their experiences in the care of patients and by patients' reporting of their experiences to nurses. Clinical scholarship is grounded in the vast array of facts and generalizations that nurses have gleaned from their clinical practice. Nurses have known and learned from many patients through actual case studies, and this knowledge has granted them a special knowledge that needs to be more systematically analyzed. The results of these analyses could serve to stimulate increased intellectual activity that could result in descriptions and classifications of nursing actions and measurement of the effects or outcomes of nursing care on patient responses. Nurses need to document this clinical knowledge in published case studies.

Consider how many nursing interventions classified as psychosocial have been described in the literature as nursing actions. Oiler and Munhall (1989) described the intervention of reassurance in a phenomenological study. Moreover, little attention has been given to studies of physical nursing care, such as the bath. There are few studies that examine the effects of bathing or massage on patient responses. More studies need to be conducted on basic nursing interventions, such as the bath, listening, comforting, providing reassurance, and using touch.

The "bright future of nursing science is at the cusp of the 21st century" and will be increasingly inspired by patient and client needs. Descriptive research on clinical interventions will be valued even more than presently and will provide an empirical base for various nursing treatments, pain management in children, coping and management of chronic illness, and nursing management of the array of symptoms reported by patients with cancer.

SUPPORT YOUR LOCAL NURSE RESEARCHER AND MAKE A LEARNING LEAP

Money is available on the federal level to nourish selected nurse researchers' research agendas, but there is also a great deal of competition. Given that a few will obtain funding through NIH/NCNR, nurse researchers must look around for other funding opportunities. Nurse researchers need funding because many nursing service organizations have not been able to budget dollars for nursing research. Few hospitals pay salaries to nurse researchers, and fewer still provide secretarial support, capital expenditures such as computers, funds for data entry and statistical support, or budget for xerox and mailings associated with a thriving nursing research enterprise. For some hospitals or other health care agencies, it may be necessary to budget for consultant fees for a nurse researcher to come in routinely to help nursing research get started in a health care agency. They may not be able to afford a part-time or full-time nurse researcher. Funding a nurse researcher to help them start a research project may help the institution in return. By helping the investigator gain access to subjects, or collecting data, and actively contributing to the dissemination of research data, may not only support the investigator but make possible to learn a great deal about how to conduct a research study. This process will market the products of the research effort and the public will be aware of what kind of interests nurses have.

Nurses need to make learning leaps and expand their education beyond associate and baccalaureate degrees, especially through research. It is estimated that there will be a deficiency of 600,000 baccalaureate degrees and excesses of 200,000 associate degree and licensed practical nurses respectively. These individuals need to become competent in research in order to be careful data collectors and effective critics of the increasing amount of published nursing research. Applying this knowledge, the patient care may improve. In the future, development educators will be teaching basis research concepts to staff, particularly to those who may not have had research courses in the past.

ETHICAL CARE AT THE END OF LIFE: REVELATIONS ABOUT WHAT NURSES VALUE

Nurses share with other care givers the commitment to help people live. They have been constantly preoccupied by the many chronically ill patients who survive acute illnesses, make tangible gains during rehabilitation efforts, and go on to lead lives that are pleasant and productive. Their knowledge of the patients who survive with difficulty, assisted by the marvels of high technological care is important. In these patients, the care/cure dichotomy prevails. Humanistic care suffers while cure is sought through seemingly futile efforts. While nurses have become expert users of health care technology and consequently participate in the advantages that technology brings to patient care, they also confront the disadvantages of the invasion that instrumentation and pharmaceuticals represent.

Nurses may note that there are many interests to be served as terminally ill patients are kept alive. Some wish that family members have enough time to prepare for their relatives' deaths, others are interested in obtaining organs to donate to transplant candidates, still others wish them to stay alive because they have a life at all costs approach to care or may not have resolved their personal attitudes about death.

It is generally acknowledged that nurses and other providers feel like failures when death comes, since they expended a lot of energy fighting it. In addition, they may practice nursing and medicine defensively when caring for patients since they fear malpractice suits. They are aware of the somewhat assaultive interventions that keep terminally ill patients alive.

Many nurses have not yet come to terms regarding how patients should die, but they acknowledge that they are often pleased when patients have a peaceful death in the presence of loved ones. Nurses often witness less than peaceful, and even uncomfortable deaths. Some nurses are better able to cope with this process. They consult with patients, relatives, friends, physicians, and other nurses in order to keep patients' and relatives' wishes in the forefront. Some strategies that can be used include: (1) initiate discussions with physicians and lobby for a team approach, (2) quote that patient's statement of his or her wishes in the chart, (3) discuss with all involved, and include the ethics committee in the discussion. Nurses will be confronted with increased numbers of complex ethical problems. They should consult the nurse ethicists of the future.

CHRONIC ILLNESS AND NINETYSOMETHING

It has become increasingly evident that lengthened life spans and widespread chronic illness and disability are the future of health care. The evidence overwhelms health care providers, and is already giving them a great deal of ideas for being able to deal directly with these trends. They are acutely aware that chronic illness care lacks the dazzle of high technological care. Many have expressed the fact that, there have been too few geriatric and rehabilitation specialists in nursing and medicine. High tech care charms neophyte clinicians, even though a few choose gerontology and rehabilitation early in their careers.

Jennings, et al. stated that "the special nature of chronic care will test the character of American society." According to these authors, the experience of chronic illness calls for scrutiny of social support systems, evaluation of coping abilities, assessment of performance of activities of daily living, and maintenance of independence and a sense of self-worth. They also project an elderly boom for 2020, a chronic care avalanche, that will force nursing and medicine away from acute care toward chronic care.

The burdens of illness will again fall on low income elderly, medically indigent, women, the working poor, and minority groups. Nurses will again face the challenges that chronic illness care brings. More will seek out the special knowledge of gerontological nursing and deal with the special concerns of the chronically ill of all ages.

NURSES AND SOCIAL POLICY FORMULATION

Social policies on poverty, housing, employment, and education affect the health of the nation. Health policy, a specific type of social policy, more directly influences the people's health. Nurses are becoming more aware of their responsibility to shape health policy and general social policy.

Members of the American Academy of Nursing have attempted to influence the shape of new health policies and to call for radical revisions of existing ones. They plan to target their efforts at health policy reform toward a more equitable, compassionate system of health care delivery. Nurses call for discussions that go "beyond the boundaries of any one profession or any one population group."

There are suggestions that health and social policies should treat the person as part of the community, the world, and the ecosystem. Nurses can position themselves to influence legislators and creators of health policy through expert testimony because of their special knowledge of health issues. Cross specialty and multidisciplinary collaboration on social policies will help the nation to stay on an intelligent course of action in the development of broad public policy.

SPEAKING WITH CLARITY AND PRIDE FOR IMPROVING THE IMAGE OF NURSING

Even though nurses have been more self-conscious in the last decade about their personal and corporate image, the public's notion of what the role of the nurse encompasses and what functions nurses perform is still controversial. Nurses in the nineties should be encouraged to identify themselves as nurses to the patients for whom they care. There is also a need to promote recent nursing activities and accomplishments to the nursing and the hospital newsletter. A continued effort to write stories on health issues for local newspapers is also encouraged. Nurses need to continue to watch the media so that unacceptable images of nurses are removed from television and movies.

MOVING TOWARD A MODEL OF PROFESSIONAL PRACTICE: A MOMENT TO MARVEL

In 1990, Newman proposed that nursing has suffered professionally because of an ineffective professional practice model. The author suggested that nursing has been slow to create a truly professional model, lacking of specificity in level of education for practice roles. The author shares many nurses' concerns that lack of differentiation among practice roles is muddied due to various entry level programs.

No one denies that the three different educational programs that lead to the licensed registered nurse classification confuses potential students and the public. Many agree that this variety in basic preparation is one of the most difficult, divisive issues the profession has faced. In health care agencies, such as hospitals, nursing personnel with different job titles work well together in spite of the differences. However, practitioners with different levels of preparation should be doing different, interrelated things. There is a need toward an integrative stage in which practice dictated by the medical paradigm and slavish devotion to technology will be replaced by a nursing paradigm that is person-centered. In this stage, education will be university based. A tri-level model of professional practice in which post-baccalaureate, baccalaureate, and associate degree/diploma nurses has been designed clarity about their practical structure and role responsibilities.

These proposals may or may not be in place by the year 2000. However, if the issues are correctly identified, and better tackled, the problems associated with the discord related to educational preparation may be resolved. Perhaps a professional model will emerge when our clinical practice is led a greater number of post-baccalaureate nurses.

HEALTHY PEOPLE 2000: NATIONAL HEALTH PROMOTION AND DISEASE PREVENTION OBJECTIVES

According to the Healthy People 2000 report, presented by the Assistant Secretary of Health, Department of Health and Human Services, Public Health Service in 1990, the nation can no longer afford not to invest in prevention. In this report, health promotion and disease prevention are touted as opportunities to use our resources more effectively. Americans will need to develop more responsible behavior and adopt healthy lifestyles; this will save the nation health care costs. The malleable factors that can be changed and are associated with such diseases as heart disease, cancer, stroke, alcoholism, HIV infection, and drug abuse can be modified.

The goals of Healthy People 2000 include: increasing the span of healthy life for Americans; reducing health disparities among Americans; and achieving access to preventive services for all Americans. With these goals in mind, nurses are in an ideal position to use their knowledge of behavioral science to help people achieve change. Some faculty are building nursing curricula on these objectives while others are targeting their research to address them. Furthermore, increased access to health care can be provided by nurses, who outnumber other health care providers and who perform health promotion activities as well. Nurses can also act as advocates for American minorities.

THE PERILS OF PLANNING FOR THE FUTURE

Nurses see the future as a challenge, but they must determine what society needs and expects from them. The society's vision of nursing may have not changed much over the past century. Tomorrow's visions will be increasingly shaped by economic realities and awareness of the forces of social change.

Nurses should construct the future to match the vision of what nursing can be and wants to be. The only peril in planning the future is for nursing not to seek what it has always sought for its clients, i.e., compassionate care that respects individual dignity and autonomy. The future of nursing is undoubtedly based on a caring health care delivery system.

ACKNOWLEDGMENTS

Subtitles were adapted from the special issue of TIME Magazine: Beyond the Year 2000: What to expect in the new millennium. 1992;140(27).

SUGGESTED READING

Anderson P: Nurse. St. Martin's Press, New York, NY, 1978.

Anderson P: Children's Hospital. Harper & Row, New York, NY, 1985.

Lindeman, McAthie M: Nursing Trends and Issues, pp. 480-487. Ashley JA: Hospitals, paternalism, and the role of the nurse. New York: Teachers College Press, 1976.

Chin PL: Preface. In Chin PL. Health Policy: Who Cares? Kansas City, MI: American Academy of Nursing, 1991.

Courter G: The Midwife. Penguin Books, New York, NY, 1981.

Dugan AB: Expanding nursing's practice terrain: imperatives for future viability. Public Health Nursing, 1985;2(1):23-32.

Fagin C: The visible problems of an "invisible" profession: the crisis and challenge for nursing. ANNA, 1988;15(2):104-109.

Fagin C: Collaboration between nurses and physicians: no longer a choice. Nursing and Health Care, 1992;13(7):354-363.

Gino C: The Nurses's Story. Bantam Books, New York, NY, 1982.

Heron E: Intensive Care: The Story of a Nurse. Ivy Books, New York, NY, 1987.

Holt FM: Speak with clarity and pride to improve the image of nursing. Clinical Nurse Specialist, 1989;3(3):126-127.

Holt V: Secret for a Nightingale. Doubleday, Garden City, NY, 1986.

Jennings B, Callahan D, Caplan AL: Ethical challenges of chronic illness. Hastings Center Report, 1988:1-16.

Malloy C, Donahue FT: Collaboration projects between nursing education and nursing service: A case study. Nurse Education Today, 1989;9:368-377.

Mauksch IG: Understanding our past to build our future. ONF, 1989;16(4):483-487.

Melosh B: The Physician's Hand. Temple University Press, Philadelphia, PA, 1982.

Newman MA: Toward an integrative model of professional practice. Profess Nurs, 1990;6(3):167-173.

Oiler C, Munhall PL: A qualitative investigation of reassurance. Holistic Nursing Practice, 1989:61-69.

Public Health Service. Healthy People 2000: National Health Promotion and Disease Prevention Objectives. Government Printing Office, Washington, DC, 1990.

Reverby S: Ordered to Care. Cambridge University Press, New York, NY, 1987.

Swackhamer A, Moss R: Caring. Berkley Books, New York, NY, 1987.

Shaver JLF: The researcher as entrepreneur and marketer. ANA Council Perspectives. ANA Council Perspectives, 1992;1(2):1-10.

Woods NF: Foreword. In Chinn PL (Ed.). Health policy: Who cares? American Academy of Nursing, Kansas City, MI, 1991.

CONTRIBUTORS

Colin E. M. Braithwaite, M.D.
Associate Professor of Surgery
University of Medicine and
    Dentistry of New Jersey
Robert Wood Johnson Medical
    School at Camden
Cooper Hospital/University
    Medical Center
Camden, NJ

John F. Byrnes, Jr., PA-C
Surgical Assisting
Southeastern Clinical Services
Orlando, FL

Aurel C. Cernaianu, M.D
Associate Professor Surgery
University of Medicine and
    Dentistry of New Jersey
Robert Wood Johnson Medical
    School at Camden
Director of Research Programs
Cooper Hospital/University
    Medical Center
Camden, NJ

Brian J. Daley, M.D.
Trauma Fellow
University of Medicine and
    Dentistry of New Jersey
Robert Wood Johnson Medical
    School at Camden
Cooper Hospital/University
    Medical Center
Camden, NJ

Anthony J. DelRossi, M.D.
Professor of Surgery
University of Medicine and
    Dentistry of New Jersey
Robert Wood Johnson Medical
    School at Camden
Chairman, Department of Surgery
Head, Division of Cardiothoracic
    Surgery
Cooper Hospital/University
    Medical Center
Camden, NJ

Stanley J. Dudrick, M.D.
Clinical Professor of Surgery
The University of Texas
Health Science Center at Houston
Surgeon-in-Chief
Hermann Hospital
Houston, TX

Bruce M. Friedman, M.D.
Assistant Professor of Medicine
    and Anesthesia
University of Medicine and
    Dentistry of New Jersey
Robert Wood Johnson Medical
    School at Camden
Director, Nutrition Support Services
Cooper Hospital/University
    Medical Center
Camden, NJ

Donald E. Fry, M.D.
Professor and Chairman,
    Department of Surgery
University of New Mexico School of
    Medicine
Albuquerque, NM

T. James Gallagher, M.D.
Professor of Anesthesiology and
    Surgery
Chief, Critical Care Medicine
University of Florida College of
    Medicine
Shands Hospital
Gainesville, FL

Linda A. Garry, PA-C
Physician Assistant
Department of Surgery
University of Medicine and
    Dentistry of New Jersey
Robert Wood Johnson Medical
    School at Camden
Cooper Hospital/University
    Medical Center
Camden, NJ

David R. Gerber, M.D.
Assistant Professor of Medicine
    and Anesthesia
University of Medicine and
    Dentistry of New Jersey
Robert Wood Johnson Medical
    School at Camden
Cooper Hospital/University
    Medical Center
Camden, NJ

Lawrence T. Goodnough, M.D.
Associate Professor of Medicine
    and Pathology
Washington University School of
    Medicine
Director, Transfusion Services
Barnes Hospital
St. Louis, MO

David R. Knighton, M.D.
Medical Director
Institute for Reparative Medicine
St. Louis Park, MN

Mary C. McCarthy, M.D.
Associate Professor of Surgery
Wright State University
Trauma Director
Miami Valley Hospital
Dayton, OH

Alan D. Miranda, M.D.
Fellow, Critical Care Medicine
Division of Pulmonary and Critical
    Care Medicine
University of Medicine and
    Dentistry of New Jersey
Robert Wood Johnson Medical
    School at Camden
Cooper Hospital/University
    Medical Center
Camden, NJ

Anthony J. Mure, M.D.
Associate Professor of Surgery
University of Medicine and
    Dentistry of New Jersey
Robert Wood Johnson Medical
    School at Camden
Cooper Hospital/University
    Medical Center
Camden, NJ

Loren D. Nelson, M.D.
Associate Professor of Surgery and
    Anesthesiology
Director of Surgical Critical Care
    Service
Vanderbilt University Medical
    Center
Nashville, TN 37232

Keith F. O'Malley, M.D.
Associate Professor of Surgery
University of Medicine and
    Dentistry of New Jersey
Robert Wood Johnson Medical
    School at Camden
Department of Surgery
Cooper Hospital/University
    Medical Center
Camden, NJ

Debra L. Priore, PA-C
Physician Assistant
Division of Cardiothoracic Surgery
University of Medicine and
   Dentistry of New Jersey
Robert Wood Johnson Medical
   School at Camden
Cooper Hospital/University
   Medical Center
Camden, NJ

Zane Robinson-Wolf, Ph.D., R.N.
Professor of Nursing
Associate Director of Nursing
   Research
Albert Einstein Medical Center
Lasalle University
Philadelphia, PA

Steven E. Ross, M.D.
Associate Professor of Surgery
University of Medicine and
   Dentistry of New Jersey
Robert Wood Johnson Medical
   School at Camden
Head, Division of Trauma
Cooper Hospital/University
   Medical Center
Camden, NJ

Alex G. Shulman, M.D.
Director, Lechtenstein Hernia
   Institute
Los Angeles, CA

Gus J. Slotman, M.D.
Associate Professor of Surgery
Head Division of Surgical Critical
   Care
University of Medicine and
   Dentistry of New Jersey
Robert Wood Johnson Medical
   School at Camden
Department of Surgery
Cooper Hospital/University
   Medical Center
Camden, NJ

Richard K. Spence, M.D.
Professor of Surgery
University of Medicine and
   Dentistry of New Jersey
Robert Wood Johnson Medical
   School at Camden
Head, Section of Vascular Surgery
Cooper Hospital/University
   Medical Center
Camden, NJ

Linda Stehling, M.D.
Director of Medical Affairs
Blood Systems, Inc.
Scottsdale, AZ

Jacqueline D. Sutton, Pharm.D.
Assistant Director Clinical Services
University of Medicine and
   Dentistry of New Jersey
Robert Wood Johnson Medical
   School at Camden
Cooper Hospital/University
   Medical Center
Camden, NJ

Philip C. Wry, M.D.
Assistant Professor of Surgery
University of Medicine and
   Dentistry of New Jersey
Robert Wood Johnson Medical
   School at Camden
Cooper Hospital/University
   Medical Center
Camden, NJ

INDEX

Abdominal
    paracentesis, 159
    trauma, 159
ABO compatibility matching, 133
Acetylcystine, 65
Acute normovolemic hemodilution, 137
Acyclovir, 85
Adrenocorticotrophic hormones, 3
Adult respiratory distress syndrome, 72
Afterload, 113
Albumin, 3, 108, 161
Allergen, 105
Allogeneic blood transfusions, 124, 127,
    140
Aminopenicillins, 83
Amphotericin B, 85, 86
Amputation, 20
Anaerobic, 78, 83
    metabolism, 115, 117
    threshold, 56
Anaphylaxis, 53
Anemia, 5
Angiogenesis, 15, 16
Angioscopy, 150
Antibacterial agents, 83
Antibiotic, 27, 78, 79
    monitoring, 86
    selection, 81
    prophylaxis, 80
Antibodies,
    IgA, 165
    IgM, 72
Anticoagulants, 106
Antiendotoxin antibodies, 72, 73
Antifungals, 85
Antioxidant, 171, 172
Antiproteases, 65
Antipseudomonal penicillins, 83, 86
Antipsychotics, 79
Antiseptics, 78
Antivirals, 85
Aortic cross-clamping, 91
Arachidonic acid, 54, 71, 167

ARDS, 63
Arginine, 6, 55, 168
Arterial oxygen content, 56, 114
Arteriograms, 20
Ascorbic acid, 8
Aspirin, 132
Atherectomy, 147
Atherosclerotic vascular disease, 146
Auth rotary atherectomy device, 147
Autocrine, 15
Autologous blood, 124, 125, 127
Azithromycin, 83
Aztreonam, 83

B-Complex vitamins, 9
B. fragilis, 83
Bacteria
    classification, 81
    contaminants, 14, 26
    endocarditis, 79, 80
    permeability, 55
    translocation, 165, 167
Bactericidal, 83
Balloon angioplasty, 145
Below-the-knee amputation, 20
Bleeding time, 133
Blood
    volume, 4
    pressure, 111
Bradykinin, 13
Branch chain amino acids, 167, 168

C. difficile, 83, 86
Calcium, 155
Capillary
    integrity, 65
    leak, 65
    permeability, 64
Carbapenems, 83
Carbohydrate, 5, 8
Cardiac
    edema, 56
    index, 112

Cardiac (*cont.*)
　　output, 55, 64, 67, 112, 113, 114
　　preload, 112
　　tamponade, 91
　　work, 67
Catabolism, 4
Catalase, 55, 65
Catheter-over-needle technique, 162
Cefotetan, 83
Cefoxitin, 83
Cell
　　damage, 56
　　debris, 14
　　lysis, 54, 57
　　proliferation, 16
Cellulitis, 53
Cephalosporin, 83, 85
Chemoattractants, 15, 26, 28
Chemotactic molecule, 16
Chloramphenicol, 86
Chlorhexidine, 78
Chloride, 66
Chronic shock, 96
Ciprofloxacin, 83
Clarithromycin, 83
Clindamycin, 85
Coagulation, 135, 166
Coagulopathy, 106, 134, 135, 159
Collagen, 5, 6,8, 16, 25, 28
Colloid, 91, 108, 109, 138, 139
Complement,
　　activation, 13, 54, 65
　　cascades, 166
Component therapy, 131
Congestive heart failure, 17
Connective tissue, 3
Consumption coagulopathy, 107
Contamination, 27
Corticosteroids, 51, 65, 73
Critical balances, 116
Crush injuries, 53
Cryoprecipitate, 107, 134
Crystalloid, 103, 105, 108, 109.138, 139
Cyclooxygenase inhibitors, 65
Cysteine, 6
Cystine, 3
Cytokine, 2, 53, 54, 64, 73
Cytomegalovirus, 85

Dazosiben, 72
Delayed hypersensitivity, 5
Delayed wound repair, 13
Dexamethasone, 71
Diabetic mellitus, 20
Diapedesis, 26
Diaphragm, 57
DIC, 159
Digestive enzymes, 28
Diltiazem, 67

Dilutional thrombocytopenia, 106
Disulfiram-like reaction, 86
Drug interactions, 86

Eicosanoids, 66
End-diastolic pressure, 112
End-diastolic volume, 56, 112
End-organ
　　dysfunction, 72
　　failure, 71
　　perfusion, 110
Endocarditis, 53
Endorphins, 167
Endothelial
　　activation, 65
　　adhesion molecule, 54
　　cell migration, 17
　　derived relaxing factor, 54
　　relaxant factor, 66
Endotoxemia, 64
Endotoxin, 53, 65
Endovascular surgery, 145
Energy requirements, 8
Enteral feeding, 92
Enteroenteral fistulas, 7
Enzymatic digestion, 26
Epidermal growth factor, 14, 15, 16
Epigastric vessels, 42
Epithelialization, 15, 18, 28
Erythromycin, 83
Erythropoietin, 126
Ethanol, 156
Exogenous amino acids, 5
Exotoxins, 53
External oblique aponeurosis, 39, 42
Extracellular matrix synthesis, 17
Extravascular lung water, 64
Exudate, 161

Factor VIII, 107, 134
Factor XII, 13
Factors, 15
Fascia transversalis, 41
Fat metabolism, 8
Femoral hernia, 43
FFP, 104, 134, 159
Fibrin
　　glue, 134
　　matrix, 26, 28
Fibrinogen, 107, 134
Fibrinolysis, 159
Fibroblast, 25, 29
　　proliferation, 6
Fibronectin, 14
Fibroplasia, 1, 2,15
Fick equation, 114
Flow-directed pulmonary artery catheter, 118
Fluconazole, 70, 71, 85

Flucytosine, 85
Fluid
　retention, 5
　replacement, 103
　challenge, 118
Fluoromisonidazole, 57
Fluoroquinolones, 83, 86
Foscarnet/ganciclovir, 85
Fractional residual capacity, 63
Fresh frozen plasma, 105, 106, 133
Fungi, 53

Gamma interferon, 54
Gastrocnemius, 57
Gastroenterostomy, 2
Genitofemoral, 42
Genitofemoral nerve, 42, 43
Glucocorticoids, 167
Glucose 6-phosphate dehydrogenase, 82
Glutamine, 169
Glycosaminoglycans, 16
Graft rejection, 53
Granules, 13
　azurophilic, 55
Growth factors, 13, 14, 26, 172

Heat stroke, 53
Hematopoiesis, 4,
Hemodilution, 138
Hemolysins, 53
Hemolytic reactions, 105
Hemorrhagic shock, 52, 90
Hemostasis, 25, 26
Hepatic clearance, 54
Hepatitis, 134
Hernial sac, 34
Herpes simplex virus, 85
Hetastarch, 66
Hip replacement, 6
Histamine, 55
Histotoxic injury, 57
Host defense, 25
Hydration, 4
Hydrogen peroxide, 54
Hydrolases, 28
Hydrophilic enzymes, 27
Hydrostatic pulmonary edema, 107, 108
Hydroxyl radicals, 54
Hydroxyproline, 6
Hyperalimentation, 4, 7
Hypertonic saline, 91, 109
Hypoalbuminemia, 2
Hypocalcemia, 153
Hypomagnesemia, 154, 155, 156
Hypoproteinemia, 2, 4
Hypoprothrombinemia, 86
Hypotension, 55, 64, 66
Hypothermia, 134, 135
Hypovolemic shock, 107, 109, 111

IgM anti-endotoxin antibody, 72
IL-2, 167
Iliohypogastric, 42
Ilioinguinal nerve, 43
Imipenem/cilastatin, 83, 86
Immune
　dysfunction, 166
　mediated organ injury, 52, 53, 105
　status, 10
Immunocompetence, 6
Immunosuppression, 105, 167
Infection, 5
　site of, 81
　types of, 77
Inflammatory
　diseases, 51
　proteins, 25
　response, 27
Inguinal
　canal, 42
　hernia, 33
Inotropes, 52, 67
Insulin-like growth factor, 15, 172
Integrins, 54
Interleukin, 26
Interleukin-1, 54, 73, 166
Interleukin-6, 57, 166
Internal oblique muscle, 46
Internal ring, 39, 43
Interstitial volume, 109
Intra-abdominal pressure, 39
Intracellular adhesion molecule-1, 54
Intraoperative blood recovery, 140
Intravascular fluid overload, 107
Intravascular volume, 110, 111
Iron stores, 126
Ischemic myocardial dysfunction, 56
Isotonic solutions, 109
Itraconazole, 85

J5 Antiserum, 72

Keratinocytes, 16
Ketoconazole, 70, 72, 73, 85
Kinin, 13, 57, 100, 116, 117

Lactic acidosis, 52, 57, 118
Laser angioplasty, 146
Leakage, 14
Leukocidin, 53
Leukotriene, 54, 65, 73
Limb salvage, 20
Lipid A, 55
Lipid moiety, 64
Lipopolysaccharide, 53, 54
Lipoxygenase, 65, 72
Lysosomal enzymes, 27, 28, 54

Macrolides, 83
Macrophage, 53, 66, 166
Malnutrition, 4
Margination, 26
Margination, 28
Marlex® mesh, 35, 43
Mast cells, 25, 26
MAST trousers, 89
Mental status, 110
Mesenchymal precursor cells, 29
Mesenteric ischemia, 53
Mesh patch, 34, 41
Metabolic acidosis, 66
Methicillin, 86
Methionine, 6
Methylprednisolone, 71
Methylthiotetrazole, 86
Metronidazole, 85
Microthrombi, 55
Microvascular shunting, 57
Mitogen, 16
Mixed venous oxygen saturation, 56, 115, 116, 118
Mixed venous oxygen tension, 115
Monobactams, 83
Monoclonal antibody, 64
Monocytes, 13,
MSOF, 53, 63, 92, 167
Multitrauma, 52
Myeloperoxidase, 54
Myocardial
    compliance, 55
    contractility, 108

Neovascularization, 2
Neuropathy, 13
Nitric oxide, 53, 55, 56
Nitrogen balance, 3
Nonhealing ulcers, 13
Nonsteroidal antiinflammatory, 132
Nosocomial infections, 77
Nuclear magnetic resonance scan, 57
Nucleotides, 171
Nutritional
    depletion, 7
    evaluation, 5
    immunomodulation, 165
    immunomodulation-combination therapy, 172
    pharmocologic agents, 167
    rehabilitation, 6
    status, 1, 6
Nystatin, 69, 70

Oliguria, 52
Oloxacin, 83
Omega-3 fatty acids, 170, 172
Omega-6 fatty acids, 170, 171, 172
Oncotic load, 105

Osmolyte HN, 172
Over-resuscitation, 104, 108
Oxidative phosphorylation, 57
Oxygen
    carrying capacity, 105, 106, 113
    consumption, 55, 56, 67, 99, 114
    delivery, 91, 92, 96, 51, 56, 67, 100, 103, 106, 113
    demand, 115
    extraction, 57, 98
    extraction ratio, 99
    free radicals, 54
    radicals, 65
    transport, 104, 110, 113, 118
    uptake, 115
    utilization, 114
    utilization coefficient, 114
Oxygen transport balance, 115

Pancreatic fistulas, 7
Pancreatitis, 52, 53
Paracrine, 15
Parenteral nutrition, 7
Penicillin
    spectrum, 84, 86
    types of, 84
Penicillinase-resistant, 83
Percutaneous transluminal angioplasty (PTA), 145
Peritoneal inflammation, 160
Peritoneal lavage, 159
PGE_1, 72
PGE_2, 167
Phagocytosis, 26
Phenotypic state, 15
Phospholipid platelet activating factor, 54
Pilonidal cysts, 3,
Plasma, 103
Plasmanate, 66
Plasmaphereses, 2
Plasmin, 13
Plasminogen activator inhibitor, 14
Platelet, 14, 106, 132
    activating factor, 65
    derived growth factor, 14, 15, 16, 18, 26
    derived wound healing formula, 18
    dysfunction, 106, 107
    factor 4, 14, 19
    transfusion, 107
    trigger, 133
Platelets, Antiaggregatory effects, 55
Polyunsaturated fatty acids, 66
Polyunsaturated fatty acids, 170
Portal hypertension, 161
Positive blood cultures, 64
Positive pressure mechanical ventilation, 112